# The Tree of Ecstasy

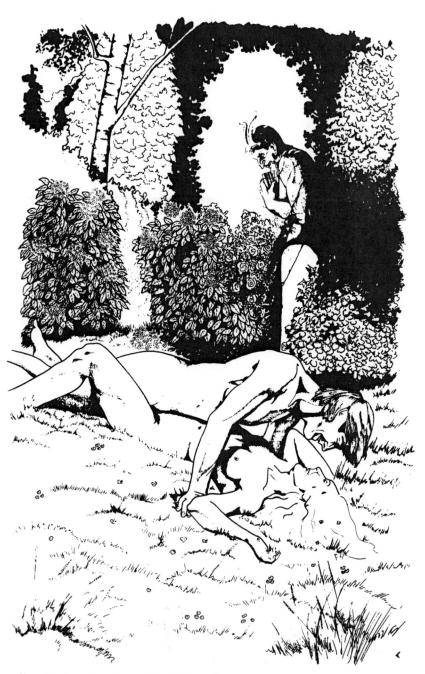

*Frontispiece:* First Love (*Paul Hardy*)

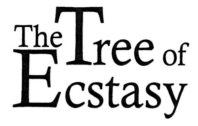

# The Tree of Ecstasy

An
Advanced
Manual of
Sexual
Magic

Dolores Ashcroft-Nowicki

SAMUEL WEISER, INC.

York Beach, Maine

First published in 1999 by
Samuel Weiser, Inc.
P. O. Box 612
York Beach, ME 03910-0612

Library of Congress Cataloging-in-Publication Data:

Ashcroft-Nowicki, Dolores.
    The tree of ecstasy: an advanced manual of sexual magic /
Dolores Ashcroft-Nowicki
        p.    cm.
    Originally published: London: Aquarian Press, 1991.
    Includes bibliographical references and index.
    ISBN 1-57863-038-X (pbk. : alk. paper)
    1. Magic. 2. Sex—Miscellanea. I. Title.
    BF1623.S4A84      1999
    133.4'3—dc21                                            98-37648
                                                                CIP

Cover illustration by Chris Hill

Printed in the United States of America
BJ

06 05 04 03 02 01 00 99
10 9 8 7 6 5 4 3 2 1

The paper used in this publication meets all the minimum requirements of the American National Standard for Permanence of Paper
for Printed Library Materials Z39.48-1984.

# Dedication

To Margaret O'Donnell and J.H. 'Herbie' Brennan, a small token of appreciation for all the laughter and good fellowship shared in Boris's room!

# CONTENTS

# ACKNOWLEDGMENTS

Quite frankly I'm amazed I found the courage to write this book! I'm even more amazed that my long-suffering publishers agreed to print it! I have no doubt that I will get denounced from the pulpit yet again, but before they drag me to the stake let me raise a glass and say, "Thank you for believing in me," and also to say a *big* thank you to Leigh Daniels and Evelyn Gauthier for the gift of "Bucky" the Apple Mac. Thanks also to John Oomkenz of Golden Lotus Products in Holland who put together a set of oils and incenses for each ritual, to Michael for his invaluable help with Chapter Two, and to Anne-Elisabeth Evason who looked after husband, house, animals, and me as I battled with the manuscript.

To those brave souls who tried the rituals and survived bloodied but unbowed, I offer my love and thanks, and if I suggest a aequel, please, talk me out of it.

My acknowledgments to Rider-Hutchinson of London and St. Martin's Press for permission to quote from W. I. Thompsons's *The Time Falling Bodies Take to Light* on page 81.

# INTRODUCTION

'Why a book on sex magic for heaven's sake?' 'You'll never get it published.' 'The Church will eat you alive.' 'Watch out for Mary Whitehouse,' (tongue firmly in cheek). 'Can I have a copy ?' 'You wouldn't *dare*.' 'What about AIDS?' All the above have been said to me and more since I decided to write this book, and the answers are as follows:

    a) Because there is a place for sex in magic when used with discretion and discrimination, and I'm fed up with it being swept under the magical carpet.
    b) I did.
    c) It makes a change from the lions eating the Christians, and anyway, they need to have something to complain about.
    d) I'll send her a copy.
    e) No, you can buy it when it comes out.
    f) Oh yes I would.
    g) I have not written a manual for promiscuous sex, but for bonded, loving partners who are also magicians. If people are stupid enough to want to sleep around and risk their health and their lives, they will do it with or without this book.

I have thought long and hard about writing this book and I am well aware that many people will behave like ostriches and look for the nearest piece of sand. Others will thump pulpits and trot out the old tired notions about the occult being a front for sex and perversion (and a fair number of them will maintain a subscription to *Penthouse* and/or *Playgirl*). But I am fed up to the back teeth of being told that sex is nasty and bad for my spiritual health.

Controversy is the spice of life and two of the most controversial subjects are sex and the occult: put them together and anything can and probably will happen. Sex is normal and most of us enjoy it, some more than others. For some it assumes the proportions of a nightmare because of tragic memories, rape, abuse in childhood or a strict and unloving upbringing. There are those who treat it like a packet of crisps and hand it around, but equally there are those who regard it as a supreme gift from God/Goddess. I happen to be one of them, and I also regard the art of magic as a legitimate means of communicating with, and offering worship to, the Godhead.

The manuals on offer that deal with sex magic either come to the subject from a purely Eastern viewpoint with no allowances made for the way Western minds work, or, in at least one instance, offer a technique *the authors* regard as Tantra, complete with something that comes perilously close to live-in group sex with rather dubious overtones. *This book* offers a complete set of rituals based on sexual magic. It is not for beginners or weirdos. All magic affects the endocrinal system of the body, and a student who has spent many years in magical training will have adjusted to the fluctuations that can occur in the system during ritual. Those with little or no serious training risk upsetting their systems – risks that may include temporary impotence and loss of sexual appetite.

I'm by no means saying this book is the only right way to perform sexual magic or that I am the one and only authority on the matter. What I am saying is: 'Here is a complete set of rituals with sex as a central theme. They offer nothing that is deviant, ungodly (unless you regard the missionary position as mandatory) or, to the magical mind at least, blasphemous.' I have written this book with care, with humour and with love, and have tried to make it acceptable to all but the most determined of narrow minds.

For partners, lovers, husbands and wives, people bonded together in the most intimate and magical of ways, these rituals are for you. Making love knows no age limit: an 80-year-old woman is still a 'Garment of the Goddess', a man is a God until the last flicker of admiration for a neat ankle or a pretty smile dies, i.e. when he's dead!

Many years ago I was told, 'God gave humanity the twin gifts of sex and sensuality to have children and fun.'

All I can say is, 'Thank God.'

Dolores Ashcroft-Nowicki

# Part 1

# THE HISTORY OF SEX IN MAGIC

# 1. PREHISTORIC RITUAL AND THE GREAT MOTHER

As an instinct and a means of continuing the species, sex is almost as old as the first form of life, as old as the galaxy of which we are a minute part. We might take it further and say that sex in one form or another has always been in existence, that it is the first principle: to create, to survive, to grow, to pass on the genetic substance of life and experience, and to encourage each species to evolve as far as it can. The dinosaurs and the sabre-toothed tiger didn't make it, but humanity got the hang of it pretty quickly – for them, sex worked like magic!

From early times sexual ecstasy, religion and magic have been irretrievably linked together. This is a natural linking: we eat when we are hungry and feel satisfied, we sleep when we are tired and feel pleasure when we wake refreshed, but when we come together in the sexual act we experience total physical and mental ecstasy. To align this feeling with the early Gods and to use it as a means to worship and communicate with those Gods was an obvious step. Cave paintings leave no doubt that prehistoric tribes used the sexual act in their ritual celebrations, and figurines such as 'The Venus of Willendorf' testify to their reverence for the fertility of woman and her ability to give new life. The female womb was the first, and remains for the magician the prime, example of the sacred chalice, with its implication of the communion between humanity and something much greater.

It took early man a long time before he realized it required two to bring a child to birth, as long as it took him to find out that the erect phallus, the source of so much personal pleasure, was in point of fact a highly potent and very important part of the whole fertility cycle. From this moment of realization he began to implement the swing from a matriarchal system to that of a patriarchal and moved away from the worship of the womb to that of the penis. This historic changeover is something I do not propose to spend much time on, as it has been more than adequately dealt with by other writers – Merlin Stone, for example, in her excellent book *The Ancient Mirrors of Womanhood*.

Sex and religion cannot be separated because each has its roots in the other and from them emerged the first magical rituals. For the early tribes the need for fertility was imperative, both in their women, to combat the high mortality rate, and in the herds of wild creatures that provided most of their food. The woman who was exceptionally fertile was regarded with awe, and was seen as being someone with special powers, highly favoured by whatever magical being it was that caused her to give birth so often. To ancient humanity anyone who fitted their concept of an ideal man or woman was considered to be more than human and was gradually elevated to the earthly image of a God. A fertile woman with her large breasts and hips spread by continuous childbearing would have become an ideal, a copy of the Great Mother. She was the prototype priestess of the Goddess, and therefore seen by the tribe as Her earthly counterpart.

As long as she could bear children such a woman would have great power within the tribe. Evidence suggests that a successful hunter wore the horns of his kill in tribute to the animal's strength and courage. By coupling with a fertile woman immediately after the hunt, these qualities were seen as being transferred by the ritualized sex to the unborn child, who in turn was thought to inherit these special powers and was therefore capable of enriching the life of the tribe. Another belief was that the animal's sacrifice of its life to feed the tribe was rewarded by rebirth in human form. This may have been one way in which the legends of half-human, half-animal forms, such as the centaurs, entered the consciousness of humanity.

# The Horned God and the Goddess

Out of such beliefs and practices one of the earliest myths was born, that of the fertile Goddess in union with the ithyphallic hunter, the first Horned God, triumphantly wearing the horns taken from his latest kill. The more successful the tribal hunter in providing meat, the greater his status within his peer group, the more likely he would be the one chosen to impregnate the 'Mother' and provide her with sexual pleasure until the next big hunt.

These celebrations would have occurred at the spring gathering of the herds to drop their young and again in the late summer when they gathered prior to migration. Therefore a hunt lasting many days and involving every man who could hold a spear would have been a half-yearly ritual. The first hunt would feed the starving tribe after the long cold months, the second would enable them stock up on food before the next winter began.

A clever and powerful woman in control of her feminine intuition would have made it her business to influence the outcome of the hunt by the promise of her sexual favours to the most successful male. Emboldened by such a promise, the men would have felt almost invincible as they set out and this would have undoubtedly added to their skill and determination. Feeling themselves to be under magical protection, such a tribe would have grown fast in numbers, eaten well, and lived longer, giving further proof, if they needed it, of the benevolence of the Great Mother.

In order to provide encouragement to the other hunters, the union would probably have been a public rite, watched by the whole group – something we would now find repugnant but which has been customary in many cultures. While the unsuccessful hunters looked on in envy, the older men would have told wild stories about their own vanished prowess, and the young girls and the boys not yet old enough to hunt would have been encouraged to look forward to their own first mating.

The chosen man would have been greatly envied and the others would have striven to outmatch his hunting skills in order to take his place with the Mother at the next big ceremony. Competition and rivalry amongst the men would have been very fierce, inevitably leading to fighting between them. In later civilizations, such fights would have become games of physical skill – wrestling, running, feats of strength, etc – and would have provided the populace with entertainment and the high priestess with the best genes for the expected child of the union.

As the chosen woman got older and did not bear so frequently or so easily, she would eventually have to choose a younger woman to take her place. The older, wiser woman would have installed her successor with chanted words, circled steps, and the shaking of bones and seed-filled gourds, for highly elaborate rituals would not yet have been devised. She would have retained her influence over the girl for a long time, perhaps until her death, which would have been seen as a return to the Goddess.

# Sacred Prostitution Cultures of the Mediterranean

If we now move on to the beginning of recorded history in places such as Mesopotamia and Chaldea, we find humanity living in agricultural groups, mostly small villages and towns but some in larger city states. The people are now divided into well-defined groups: artisans, workers, slaves, officials, warriors, rulers, and priests. There are laws, markets, temples, and even the beginnings of a monetary system as well as a fairly sophisticated system of education for the ruling class. Already the earlier myths and legends surrounding the Goddess and Her Consort would have been considered ancient and set in times long ago. But the tribal Mother and the hunters whose prowess she rewarded lingered on. In the temples, among the priests and priestesses, there would have been the *Hierodules* who served as sexual aspects of the Goddess for the men who came to worship Her. In this era, sacred prostitution was not looked down upon, but seen as natural and holy and a service to the Goddess Herself.

To the temple a man would come with an offering for the Goddess – perhaps he wanted more children, or some extra yield from his fields, cows or camels. In lying with the priestess he would feel himself blessed and honoured. She in her role as the Goddess would listen to his prayers in the silence after their union and perhaps grant them if she was pleased with his sexual performance. It was correspondence magic pure and simple. The man would go home full of confidence, more relaxed and therefore perhaps more likely to impregnate his own wife. The new-found conviction that the Goddess had listened to him might also give him renewed strength to dig more irrigation canals and the fields would yield an increase in return.

In modern terms such priestesses would be seen as prostitutes and harlots, but in their own times they were acknowledged as a vital and important part of the temple hierarchy. In the cult of the Goddess Mylitta in Babylonia, every woman once in her life sat at the entrance to the temple and went with the first man who offered her money. This fee was then given to the temple as an offering. It was seen as the just dues required by the Goddess, which no woman would dream of denying Her.

# The Descent Myth and the Love Goddess

At certain times of the year the temples would present enactments of the old stories such as 'The Descent of Innana' where the Goddess, mourning the death of Her lover, goes down into hell to suffer loss, pain, humiliation, and even death. The Goddess of

Death demands everything She has in payment – Her jewels, clothes, crown, the magical girdle worn by all love goddesses – and finally demands Her death. When the Goddess of Love and Fertility 'dies' everything dies, so the Gods themselves petition for Her to be restored to life. She emerges from the Land of the Dead with Her lover and the earth comes alive again. This was celebrated every year and bears a remarkable resemblance to our own Easter celebrations, with its emphasis on the death and resurrection of a God – except that the ancient enactment ended with a public act of sex. This was to reassure the people that the Goddess of Love and Fertility was truly restored to them, and that She and Her lover were capable of copulation, thus ensuring that the earth would yield a harvest. In the earliest times the ritual would always have been in full view of the people but gradually it became more withdrawn. Finally only the high priest and/or the high priestess would have been present during the final part of the ritual.

# The Sacrificed King

About this time another ancient belief had its beginnings, that of a magical link between the king and the land. As long as the king was fertile and *seen* to be fertile the land would yield, if not then only the shedding of his blood would suffice. But such a ritual worked only with the aid and consent of the Goddess, either in the person of the high priestess or that of the queen, *for She was the land*.

From this basic premise many similar myths have emerged: the corn king, such as Osiris, cut down to rise again; the oak king of the sacred grove, doomed to fight all comers until one should defeat him and take his place. There are the harvest lords, John Barleycorn, the Lammas King, all destined to die for the land and rise again. Always the cause of the king's death, and sometimes his executioner, was the Goddess, and the penultimate act of the tragedy was the coupling of the Goddess and the king, for his seed had to be left in Her womb to provide him with a new incarnation.

# Woman as Enroyaler of Kings and Source of Inspiration

In Egypt the bloodline of the royal family was kept as pure as possible by inbreeding, something which eventually led to genetic disaster. The old tradition of the woman symbolizing the power, fertility, and persona of the earth and the Goddess of the Earth was very strong here. For a new pharaoh to rule he had to marry the queen or the daughter of the former ruler. She may have been his mother or his sister, but nevertheless only she had the power to enroyal him and grant him the right to sit on the throne. This unwritten law is seen in action throughout history – to offer an example we need only look to the marriage of Henry Tudor to Elizabeth Plantagenet, daughter of Edward IV. As the victor of the Battle of Bosworth, where Richard III met his death, Henry became king of England by force of arms, but in order that this should be seen to be a legitimate claim (his own were on the dubious side) he married the young Elizabeth of York and through her bloodline became accepted as a true king in the eyes of the populace.

To return to Egypt, the frequently seen statues of the king in the form of the young Horus seated on the lap of Isis symbolize this enroyalment. The use of the word 'lap' has long been a euphemism for the female vulva and by 'sitting on the lap', i.e. sexually penetrating, the Goddess/royal wife, he was making a claim to the throne. Another phrase often used is that of being 'over the moon', or wildly happy and enthusiastic. But being over the moon is another synonym for intercourse, the moon being the woman lying beneath the man.

Although by now the swing to the patriarchal system was almost complete, much of the matriarchal worship survived – indeed it has never completely disappeared. Wherever it is found, sexual magic is never far away. The Goddess is, after all, not only Isis Queen of Heaven and Gaia the Earth Mother, She is and always has been Venus/Aphrodite the Goddess of Sexual Love. In many ways and under various disguises She has inspired the male of the species and coaxed the best from him throughout history. She has inspired some of the greatest of the world's paintings and sculptures, and been the focal point of the finest love poems and prose in world literature. Her triple gift of fertility, love and sexual pleasure remains the triangle on which much of our existence is built, a gift that holds for humanity the ultimate magic, recognition of the divinity of the self.

To move from Egypt to classical Greece and Rome, we immediately find that similar laws prevail: Oedipus becomes king upon his marriage with Iocasta, as does Aegistheus when he takes Clytaemnestra as a wife. Odysseus was away from his island kingdom for many years during which his son by Penelope grew to manhood, yet the son did not inherit the crown, for that would go to the man Penelope chose as her husband. This was the main reason for so many suitors clamouring at her door. Yet even a marriage ceremony does not make the suitor a king – only the first act of sex with his new wife will enroyal him.

# Sex and Ritual in Classical Greece

Almost the whole of Greek myth is to a greater or lesser extent concerned with sex. Gods and Goddesses sought out human lovers and their progeny became the demi-gods, the heroes and the women of power such as Cassandra the prophetess of Apollo, Danae, Leda, Europa, and Io, all of whom won the sexual favour of Zeus at one time or another. There was also the legendary Helen of Troy whose face 'launched a thousand ships and burned the topless towers of Illium'. These were all half-human, or made so by their interaction with a God, but Psyche, the best known, was wholly human and won her immortality by her devotion and her determination to win back her lover Eros, the God of Love himself.

The Greek idea of sex had both its light and its darker side. On the one hand it was seen as something wholly natural and certainly something to be used in ritual and worship. It was a gift from the Gods themselves and as such it was to be used and to be seen to be used and appreciated. On the other hand the Female Mysteries of Samothraki were dark and bloodstained and almost certainly involved the sacrifice of young men at one point in their history. The priestesses carried small, wickedly sharp, leaf-shaped knives as part of their ritual equipment.

Greek women had their own exclusively female rites and mysteries, mostly concerned with fertility, and sometimes with Herms or phallus-shaped stones as part of the ritual regalia. The female population of both Greece and Rome were fully conscious of their sexual appetites and were not afraid to indulge them when given the chance. Quite apart from the wives, mothers and daughters were the *Hetairai* – we would call them high-class call girls. Besides being sexually experienced, many were also highly educated, and they could and did maintain houses where men would gather to talk and discuss with them everything from art to warfare, from music to philosophy. Attended by their eunuch slaves, they graced banquets and festivals with their presence and wielded enormous influence over the men who sought their company – among whom were the very highest in the land.

There were two other groups of women in ancient Greece whose lives were given over to the practice of sex: the *Dicteriades* and the *Auletrides*. The former were bound by law to satisfy the demands of those men who visited them. They were kept apart from other women, had to wear a specific form of dress, and had no rights of citizenship. However many of them did manage to escape from this sexual slavery and even married into respectable families. The Auletrides were musicians and dancers, and the Greeks loved music. If they could sing as well they were able to command quite high payment for their services. But only the Hetairai were able to afford the large houses, slaves, and jewellery that they displayed at their banquets. With their elegance, grace and learning they were undoubtedly the equal of the men they entertained.

# Love Goddesses and Phallic Gods

All sexual magic comes under the dominance of Aphrodite, the Goddess of Love, under one or another of her many names, and in conjunction with her consort who is both son and lover. In one version of the legend she is said to have sprung from the bloodstained foam of the sea after Chronus, the God of Time and Space, had castrated his father Ouranos and flung the bleeding genitals into the ocean.

The theme of this tale is picked up again further on in time when a Tartar princess named Tamara, not wishing to become the chattel of a husband, took a new lover on the eve of each new moon, then castrated him the next morning and left him to 'water the earth with his blood'. The legend goes on to say that in the gardens of her palace, walled against the constant wind of the steppes, she grew the most delicate and tasty of fruits. No wonder, considering how her garden was watered!

But not all sexual rites were bloody and horrific – the rituals of Priapus, for example, were riotously and unabashedly erotic. Wooden phalloi of every size and description were carried in procession and figs (a symbol for the feminine vulva) were thrown into the crowd. The largest phallus of all was carried in a chariot drawn by a group of young men called the *Phallophoroi* who chanted the ancient Greek version of rugby songs as they propelled their idol around the city. On these few days of the year everyone flung caution to the winds and went on the town, and the only horrific thing about it was the hangover afterwards.

Not a great deal has survived concerning the content of the rites of Pan, one of the oldest of Greek Gods and often mistaken for Priapus, except that many of them were sexual in nature. It is very probable that they equated with those in the temple of Mendes in the Egyptian Delta. It was here that the Goat-Headed God was worshipped (Pan, you remember, is only goat-footed) for the blessing of fertility of women, fields, and animals. I have written more of this in the first ritual in Part Three, and warn readers that the Goat God of Mendes can no longer be used in safety, as its image has been too tainted for it to be used in ritual.

In contrast the Eleusian Mysteries, though very sexual in overtone, were a little more restrained. Their heyday was over by 1400 BC, but they survived into the early Christian era, though condemned utterly by the early Church Fathers, for whom any form of sexuality was obscene. Yet the innermost rituals offered to those who were admitted set out the first principles of Nature, the knowledge of creation, in fact that very same knowledge that was denied to Adam and Eve until the first bite of that fateful apple.

# Evidence of Sexual and Goddess Worship in Biblical Times

It is held by some historians that the Hebrew God Yaweh was originally a phallic deity. Indeed, the Hebrews have not always worshipped a monotheistic God, nor always a male God. Phallic stones and pillars were set up for worship in many towns and cities throughout what was then Palestine, and the Goddess Anat or Anath was an integral part of the religion of the people for many centuries. Even today, although the man is the head of the family, it is the wife and mother who guides the household and through her that the bloodline of the Jewish faith descends. If a Jewish girl marries outside her faith, her children can be counted as Jewish, but if a man marries outside his faith, it is not so straightforward. We see here the continuing 'enroyalment' by the female.

The emphasis laid on the exploits of certain women in the Bible show a clear indication of Goddess worship. One only has to read 'The Song of Deborah' (see Judges V) to realize that here was a true 'Garment of the Goddess', a warrior maid of power and courage who for a time became a ruler and a commander of the

Israelite army in her own right. The story of Susanna and the elders is another pointer: even through the distortion of centuries of mistranslation and misinterpretation it reads like a ritual. Another important 'Goddess' symbol to consider is the story of Queen Esther. If read with an understanding of the Rite of Hathor, or the Great Rite, it becomes clear that this queen was also a priestess of the Goddess and the king had reached a point in his years of rule when he had to prove his virility. And although restricted in space to devote to this subject, we cannot bypass 'The Song of Solomon', one of the most glorious love poems ever written and containing a great deal of information hidden between its lines.

# Pillars and Stones as Sexual Symbols

A great deal has been edited out of the Bible, and even more has been mistranslated. Those stories and legends reinterpreted by Robert Graves and Raphael Patai in *Hebrew Myths: The Book of Genesis* show a markedly sexual content. The worship of the phallus in the form of a stone pillar or a sacred tree has been known for thousands of years and traces of it can be found in many Bible stories. The pillar built by Jacob after his dream of the angelic ladder is one instance. The pillar of fire that went before Moses as he led the Jews out of Egypt is another. The burning bush, and the pillar of cloud that descended before the Tabernacle where Moses talked with God offer other examples. The great pillars that upheld the Temple built by Solomon were even given names, indicating that they were regarded as being more than simply stone supports for the roof. Church architecture has been following this example ever since, indeed some of the pillars of our great cathedrals are of outstanding beauty and grace. Even today we refer to a prominent male member of a congregation as 'a pillar of the church'. Old ways and beliefs die hard, and some simply transmute into a similar symbology. In modern Christian hymns God is continually referred to as a 'rock', for example 'Rock of Ages'.

Similarly, in the Bible God/Yaweh is often described in the same terms. 'Of the rock that begat thee thou art unmindful' (Deuteronomy 32:18), 'For who is God save the Lord? and who is a rock, save our God?' (2 Samuel 32) and 'To shew that the Lord is upright: he is my rock' (Psalm 62:2) are just a few examples.

The term 'rocks' or 'stones' is often used to refer to the male testicles, and from early historical times right up to the Middle

Ages oaths, promises and statements were sworn 'with a hand laid upon the sacred stone'. Sometimes instead of the word 'stone' or 'rock', the euphemism of 'the thigh' was given. When taking office, the oath of loyalty was taken with the right hand beneath the testicles of the king. A man taking a solemn and holy oath often did so with his hand holding either his testicles or his penis. In certain parts of the Middle East this custom still prevails even today.

# The Dark Ages

After the fall of Rome and with the rise of Christianity, sex began to be denied, both as a source of magical power and as a source of pleasure between two people. Whereas in the old world sex was looked on as a gift of the Gods to be used in joy and without shame, it now became a sin, a means by which the Devil (an entity unknown until then) could tempt mankind into damnation. By now it had become *man*kind, for women were regarded as evil, as temptresses who could drag men down into the pits of Hell by their wiles. The woman was totally subservient to the male: she had to wear what she was told, do what she was told, obey her father, her brother, her husband, her son, her confessor and her king. Sex was something she was punished with, and no longer shared as an equal. Her sole values were her ability to bear children and her use as a bargaining point, for she could be a bribe or a prize of war. Her pride, her womanhood and her powers were all dragged in the dust. The indignity and cruelty of things like the chastity belt were commonplace. Women often died as the result of blood poisoning caused by the wearing of such contraptions for years on end. Childbirth, malnutrition and the lack of even the simplest of hygiene gave a woman no more than 30 years of life on average. The Goddess and Her sexual magic seemed completely forgotten. Or were they?

## The Witch Cults

Though the ancient mysteries had fallen, a little of their light still burned and the last of their wisdom lay hidden in myth and legend. The old ways, fragmented and dispersed, had become the property of the common folk. Isolated in villages and farms and tiny hamlets all over Europe the old ones kept alive the flame of knowledge. Hidden within it all was the ancient knowledge concerning the power of sexual magic.

Unfortunately the knowledge was scattered: all that was left were bits and pieces, most of which were hard to understand. In the ancient mysteries the priests and priestesses had been trained and educated to understand and use the magical creative power of the male and female in union. Now it had passed in a fragmented form to the untrained and mostly uneducated. But that was enough to keep it smouldering. These people remembered the old festivals and their symbols, and some of the old chants as well, though sometimes the words were garbled. The symbols changed and overlaid each other, but they still worked.

The fertility dances and practices to make the fields and animals yield, the signs and symbols that brought man to maid, the herbs and healing plants that aided the mind and eased the body, all these were remembered. The 'witches' could no longer openly use the symbol of the phallus of the Horned God, but used instead the besom, its carved penis head hidden within the thick bundle of twigs that served as a broom. The moon cup became the cauldron, and the two together could symbolize the physical and sexual aspect of the creative power.

For a while it seemed as if the Church would let them be, but then came the Inquisition and the burning times. If the early Church Fathers had begun the attack on women and the place of sex as a legitimate means of worship, then the medieval Church took it to the ultimate cruelty. Men used their powers to humiliate and torture the Goddess in Her earthly form. Gone were the memories of the temple rites, now condemned as obscene. Young girls, mothers with children and old women were stripped, prodded and poked with impunity by men whose natural sexual desires had been warped and repressed, and they did it out of *fear* – fear of the women's powers, fear of the echoing powers they felt within themselves and had been taught were wrong and depraved. For hundreds of years the fires of shame burned and literally millions of women, children and even men were tortured to death. Their crime was to hold to an ancient way of belief for which many were willing to die and did. When Christian martyrs died for their beliefs they were pronounced 'blessed', but when a witch died for hers she was damned. All this in the name of *love* – a love that could not bear another form of itself. It was not until the so-called Age of Reason that the fires of the Inquisition died down, but the animosity towards the Mysteries remains still, just below the surface of the modern Church.

## Human Rights

Even today there is fear and condemnation of the ancient ways – the Declaration of Human Rights is quoted whenever someone feels their way of life, religion, cult or holy name has been defamed, but a witch or a pagan is denied this 'human right' to their belief and is still persecuted because the old appellation of 'devil worshipper' remains the cry of the Church. No one complains when a mosque or a Hindu temple is built in a mostly Christian community to accommodate its adherents, but let a group of those who practise the ancient ways of the Gods light a fire on a hilltop at Beltane and the locals rise in a body. No one comments in the papers when a religious procession celebrating Chinese New Year or the end of Ramadan or a festival of Ganesha passes by. However, let an *occult* group hold a festival to celebrate their beliefs and the gutter press is there, together with groups of so-called Christians walking up and down with placards denouncing something that was holy long before Christianity arose and its adherents began to burn priceless books, records and artifacts because they celebrated a way of life that was different from their own.

# The Creative Force as the Basis of all Magic

In the practice of the Western Mystery Tradition much of the ritual work is based on the correspondences of the Qabalah. The mandala or symbol of this tradition is the Tree of Life. Indeed the rituals written for this book are based on the 10 spheres of the Tree – 11 if you count the invisible sphere of Da'ath. When these are placed in position on the human body, the place of Yesod, the moon sphere, is seen as being situated on the genitals.

Yesod is the sphere of creation allied to the element of water, itself an essential for life. Its other names are 'The Foundation' and 'The Machinery of the Universe'. All this indicates that here lies the seat of creativity, the essence of life itself where first principles come into being. In short, the act of sex is that which calls life into manifestation, the creative power that underlies everything in the cosmos and created the cosmos itself.

The determination by a minority to make of humanity's sexual power something obscene and depraved, dirty and shameful, is to deny a miracle, the miracle of love between two people. Such a power, such a force is more than physical gratification: it can become a hymn, a prayer, a paean of worship and gratitude for such power. However, all power can be misused and sex is no exception. Sexual harassment is a misuse; the demanding of sexual favours in return for something badly needed is a misuse. The causing of pain, terror and humiliation in the act of rape is more than a misuse, it is a spiritual sin, the desecration of the first grail, the female womb.[1] A womb is a sacred place where the miracle of creation is enacted, or where the sacrifice of a man's seed is poured out in worship of the Goddess. In the older form of the marriage service the groom said to his bride '. . . with my body I *thee worship'*, a remnant of the ancient ways set neatly into a Christian ceremony.

## Power in Ritual

Every ritual is powered from the sexual centre, whether or not those working the ritual are aware of it. Only a very few rituals have a specifically sexual context and require the physical act, but all require fuelling through the energies of those working the ritual. Most of the time the participants are either unaware of the need to empower the work, or else do not have the required amount of trained concentration to focus their power on the intention of the rite. Those who are fully trained and can call up that inner power and hold it steady may truly call themselves magicians. The difference in the atmosphere and in the energies that fill the intention of the ritual when the officers are truly in charge of their creative powers is unmistakable.

## Creativity in Magic

There is a tendency for some magicians to hang on to outmoded and outworn rituals and the ways in which they are worked. With so much creative force inside us there is no reason at all why it should not be used. It is true that tradition is something to cherish and some of the older rituals, especially those of the Golden Dawn, can be beautiful and moving, but in my opinion and in that of many other magicians, they have had their day. By all means use them once in a while, but we are entering upon a new era and *now* is the time to create new ways of thinking, living and being. In the Yesodic centre, within The Foundation sphere, lies the power of creativity. If this is linked to the diversifying powers of Netzach, or to the intellectual powers of Hod, the influx of new ideas could be almost overwhelming in their intensity of feeling.

I often teach my students to use the triangles on the Tree – using the influence of just one sphere can be useful, using two in balance is much better, but by using three and allowing the power of two to manifest through the power of the third you are beginning to really use the Tree and your inner magical power. If you place the Tree of Life on the human figure and draw a line from Yesod to Hod across to Netzach and down again to Yesod you have the Triangle of Power, Diversity and Thought (see p.90). It is no coincidence that if we go back to those ancient figurines of the Great Mother many of them show that same triangle incised over

---

[1] See my *First Steps in Ritual* for The Reconsecration of the Womb rite (The Aquarian Press, Wellingborough, 1990).

Her genital area. The fertility of the Mother is not confined to giving birth to children of the body, but also to children of the mind. These are the spheres to use when creativity is needed. These are also the spheres to activate when power is needed for ritual of any kind.

## Using the Creative Power for Healing

There are other uses for the creative power than ritual, and healing comes high on the list, especially self-healing, which is always the most difficult. Difficult because whether we admit it or not, many of us, especially when we arrive at the point where middle age hits us below the belt, enjoy the attention our little 'troubles' bring to us. Arthritic knees may give pain and make walking trouble-some, but they also mean the younger members of the family making the tea when you mention how badly the damp weather affects your ability to get up and down. We have all been guilty of such things, so to suddenly appear beaming with health and with the constitution of an ox will certainly raise a few eyebrows. Nevertheless an ailing magician is a contradiction in terms. Even if you cannot completely cure yourself, you can use your creative power to make your quality of life a lot better.

You might say that to use the creative power in magic you need the head and the belly of the snake, i.e. the imagination and visualizing powers of the mind and the power supplied by the sex centre. Over the years I have gradually evolved my own system of combining the two. To use the power for self-healing you will need to bring it up from the moon centre and feed it into the mid-brain where the five senses pool their energies. Begin as soon as you wake up, stretch every limb and roll your head from side to side. This helps you to wake up and get everything going after resting all night. Take away your pillow, lie flat and relax. Concentrate the mind on the genital centre until you begin to feel it growing warmer. If it helps, try a little sensual visualization, but do *not* employ masturbation: you want to obtain energy not dissipate it. When you can feel the warmth filling the centre pull it upwards like a stream of warm air up the front of your body pulling it over the belly, the stomach, the chest, lungs and throat and right up to the tip of the tongue. Return your attention to the sex centre and again pull the energy up but this time up your back over the buttocks and up the spine, over the head down the nose and in through the nostrils to the roof of your mouth. (You will be doing this exercise again prior to one of the rituals, so think of this as a trial run.) Now touch the tip of your tongue to the roof of your mouth and the two meridians will unite in a warm rush of energy that fills up the mid-brain area.

You can also try another form of this exercise by pooling the

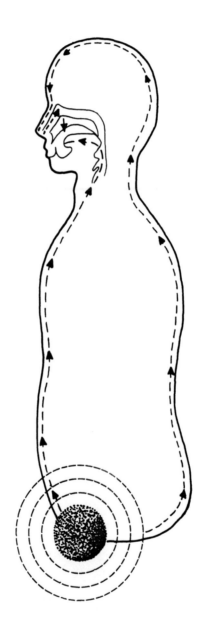

*Figure 1:* Self-healing exercise

energy in the sex centre as before but 'seeing' it flow up through the spine like a wave of red-coloured light to plug itself into the mid-brain area. Once there you can draw up as much energy as you need. Do this each morning and you will be surprised how much stronger and brighter you will feel. If you vary the colour you can also vary the use of the energy. With blue you can calm yourself down, while with green you can stimulate your creativity (this works very well because you have the creative foundation point feeding the creative receptors in the brain). Yellow, gold and deep rose will heal and work especially well after surgery. Orange is good for those who earn their living by speaking or writing: it stimulates the communication centres in the throat. Violet and indigo are for use before sleeping and can stimulate dreaming for a purpose such as untangling problems. For the initiate coming to the end of a life cycle, these last colours will also help to release the silver cord cleanly and quickly and allow the etheric to go free. You can teach others to do this for themselves but they must understand that the power used is a natural rerouting of sexual power, which by its very nature has the ability to create what the mind visualizes.

You can use this exercise in many different ways and evolve your own methods of healing and renewing yourself and others. You can use the same exercises just before the start of a ritual, but always temper the power to the need, not the other way around. Do *not* call up more power than you think you will need or the results can be chaotic as the power seeks to find a means of expression. Err on the side of too little rather than too much.

Many people ask me where I get all my energy from. How is it, they ask, that I can work with anything up to 50 people over a full day, sometimes 9 a.m. to 9 p.m., and still keep up my energy levels? Well now you know – I 'plug' in to the universal creative energy through my own energy centre. You can do the same.

# 2. LOVE IS THE FOUNDATION

'Woman,' said the philosopher Anaximander, 'is the unlimited, infinite, and containing principle of life. Man is the limited, finite, and vanishing principle.'

Without doubt women have had a raw deal over the past few thousand years. It is only in this century that they have finally laid claim to that status that was theirs in the time of the Goddess. Listen to Shakespeare's words put into the mouth of Petruchio in *The Taming of the Shrew*:

> I will be master of what is mine own;
> She is my goods, my chattels; she is my house,
> My household stuff, my field, my barn,
> My horse, my ox, my ass, my anything;
> And here she stands, touch her whoever dare.

Yet in Babylon women were regarded as equal and were paid the same in wages when they did a man's work. This has been proven by the translation of tablets found in the library of Ashurbanipal, king of Babylon.

## Ancient Laws Pertaining to Women

Would you believe that there are still places in the western world where the law of *jus prima noctis*, sometimes called *le droit de seigneur*, is still unrepealed! There are still religions teaching that a woman has no soul. In the sixth century, the Provincial Council of Macon spent weeks debating that subject, and as recently as 1895 a minister preached from the pulpit that a woman was without a soul. In England up to the end of the last century a husband had the legal right to beat his wife providing he used a stick no thicker than his thumb! In Russia a set of birch rods were part of every bride's trousseau, and these she meekly handed over to her husband as soon as they were alone after their marriage. Small wonder that the rise of the feminist movement during this century has been so swift and so determined. Sophia has risen and is demanding Her ancient rights.

## Female Mutilation
We have already discussed the cruelty of the chastity belt, but there was also the *zona virginalis*, a belt worn by every unmarried woman to indicate to all that she was unmarried. Only her husband had the right to remove it, this being done on the wedding night to symbolize the fact that he now held the right to impregnate her. Even today, when many women have won the right to lead their own lives, many young girls in the Middle East are forced to undergo the horrors of female circumcision. To their eternal shame there are doctors in London who will still perform it, their excuse being that it will at least be done under hygienic and ideal conditions. For such a practice there are *no* ideal conditions.

## Fear of the Mother Symbol
Why are such cruel practices still used against women? Mainly because of the age-old fear of the woman/Goddess and her control of life and death. The deeply-buried race memory of the sacrificed hunter and the need to accept his kingship from the Mother's hand has led to the desire to dominate and punish the Mother symbol. At the same time she is held up as an ideal of love and desire. She is the first figure a man sees at birth and often it is her name on his lips at death. This ambiguity towards the female has persisted for centuries and though we have won a lot of our power back, there is still a way to go. There is no doubt that there are women who have ruined the lives of fathers, brothers, husbands, sons and lovers, just as there are those who have been the making of them, and psychology abounds with reasons for both. But all men fear the power of women – so what is that power?

# The Power of Woman

## The Triple Power
The Goddess has three faces, and woman has three kinds of power: birth, life, and death. Each power has three levels. All are

linked together but entered upon separately and at different stages
of life. Each holds different rewards and terrors for men.

The theologians may rant and rave and quote their holy books,
but the fact remains that the first life forms to appear were female
and probably parthenogenetic. The female is the 'womb-man'
from which others of her kind emerge; the male is a mutant of the
species that came into being because evolution needed and
demanded it. That may not be palatable, but neither is it shameful
or humiliating, it is simply the way things happened. This may
come as a shock to some people, but the Bible is wrong about who
came first – still, as it is merely a pretty story it is hardly worth
getting steamed up about.

### The Power of Birth

Birth is the first female power. The female takes the seed of the
male into herself and this is his first fear, for a part of himself is
sucked into her inner darkness. This seed is alive, it contains his
own life force, the man and his seed are one. There are millions of
sperm, yet only one – or rarely more than one – will survive. To
the subconscious mind of man this makes woman a multi-murder-
ess, for the unsuccessful sperm die and become nothing. They
disappear as if they had never been and a part of the man dies
with them. Many Eastern sexual practices advocate the retention
of semen, believing its entry into the vagina shortens a man's life,
while retention will lengthen it. As each sperm is capable of
fertilization, every act of coition offers millions of permutations
that could become a child, yet only one will win the race. Nature
works along the lines of 'nothing succeeds like excess': the more
sperm, the more likely a child will come of the union. This is the
power of birth on the first level.

But birth is not always physical: ideas, thoughts, creations of
the mind all come to birth in a similar way. Men who are creative
in their work and in their life often need a woman around them,
not necessarily a wife but perhaps a mother, sister, colleague or
friend, who acts as a catalyst. The feminine power to contact the
inner levels of the cosmos is well known in occult circles. A
woman is stronger in that area just as a man is stronger physically.
Throughout history women have inspired men in the areas of
poetry, art, literature, sculpture and all facets of human existence.
Just as she takes his physical seed into her depths, so woman
takes man's needs, ideals, and desires into her psychic depths and
feeds them back to him from the higher realms. She is the Muse,
the daemon, the mirror in which he can see more clearly than by
his own efforts. Yet when his faint thoughts and tenuous ideas are
gathered up and fed into her higher, inner self, man feels as if he
has lost sight and control of them as he loses sight and control of

his seed. There is a fear that his mental children will be destroyed as well, but in the end they are returned to him enriched and completed. This is the power of birth on the second level.

As a spiritual phenomenon birth or rebirth is surprisingly common. At least one in eight people will at some time in their lives experience an inner vision of a spiritual nature. It may last a few days then fade from memory, it may last longer and change them in a small way, it can totally change them body and soul. Women cope more readily with this kind of phenomenon than men. Again, with a man, it is the feeling of being out of his own control that makes the difference. A woman, with her innate ability to touch the inner side of life, accepts it and blends her will with that of the visionary experience. For a man it is yet another temptation from an unknown source. However, when a man can accept the experience he goes into it with heart and soul and is reborn completely. The perfect example of this is seen in the life of St John of the Cross and in his beautiful 'love poetry' likening the Church to the Bride, the Beloved, and the focal point of his life. Alongside this, one has the female example of Teresa of Avila, John's lifelong friend and, on the inner levels, his true mate. The symbol of such experiences, especially those occurring within a religious atmosphere, is very often the Virgin Mary. Visions of this aspect of the Goddess have been given to many people during the last 200 years and almost always it has caused a total change in the life of that person. The power of the woman to cause spiritual change within the man can save him or damn him. This is the power of birth on the third level.

*The Power of Life*
Although there is no doubt nature has given men a stronger physical body, women cope better. Girl babies survive adverse birth traumas more readily, while women survive better in life-threatening circumstances and are less affected by cold and disease. The female was given this edge in order to ensure the survival of the species. To repopulate a devastated community only one or two healthy males are needed, so long as they are outnumbered by healthy, fertile women. In short, biologically speaking the females *must* survive in reasonable numbers, but there need only be a few males. Nature made sure of things by implanting in the male a basic urge to protect the female and her young at the cost of his own life if necessary. Deep down in the subconscious mind man knows and resents this. He feels expendable, and as far as Nature is concerned he is, almost. There is also a resentment that a woman can go on receiving pleasure in the act of sex time and time again, whereas a man, even in his sexual prime of late teens/early twenties, cannot achieve continuous

erections. Woman is a natural survivor and what is more she can be multi-orgasmic. This is the power of life on the first level.

Also, ever since the beginning of medicine, humanity has gradually extended its life expectancy. If neolithic man made it to his eighteenth birthday he was lucky, but his mate, despite the dangers of childbirth, could get to her twentieth. Century by century, discovery by discovery, medicine has pushed back the frontiers of death, fighting tooth and nail for every inch. By the end of this century men will have an average life expectancy of 78 and women will expect 82. After a race of some millions of years women are still winning. This is the power of life on the second level.

Every now and then one part of the human race seems to uproot itself and move several thousand miles to rebuild its life in a new environment. The Celts did it early on, the Aryans did it, the Phoenicians hardly put foot on land they were so busy sailing around the Mediterranean and adjacent shores. Vikings left Scandinavia and settled in Britain and northern Europe while the Portuguese and Spanish left large colonies almost everywhere, having slaughtered most of the original inhabitants. By the eighteenth century the New World was opening up and Australia was looming on the horizon, then finally in the 1800s came the great rush from all parts of the world to America, the land of opportunity, almost totally wiping out the American Indian in the process.

Families headed to America for many reasons – to evade religious and political persecution or poverty; out of a desire for adventure, a new horizon, or a few acres of land for their very own. At the heart of every family that arrived were the women. Most came because they were told they were coming by their menfolk. They were uprooted, taken from everything they knew and loved, and arrived knowing nothing of the land, its language, culture or laws. Some came carrying little boxes of earth from 'the old country', some came fiercely determined that their children and grandchildren would have opportunities denied to them. Women who had lived on farms and in small villages lived in cramped tenements and worked in sweat shops for a few pence. Later many of them moved on, crossing a virtually unknown country with every kind of hazard from snakes to hostile tribes, from cholera to impassable mountain ranges. They broke new land and planted corn, learned to ride a horse and shoot a gun. They followed their menfolk to Alaska and the gold mines, and to Texas and blistering heat. And they survived – they sometimes lost their homes, their looks, their children, their husbands and their faith, but they survived more often than the men because they adapted to the conditions that prevailed. The ability to adapt is the power of life on the third level.

## The Power of Death

In giving birth to a new life, woman also gives death, for we begin to die as soon as we are born. We spend our whole lives moving slowly but surely towards an unknown destination about which we know nothing and can never know anything until we arrive. Love, sex, marriage, pregnancy and birth, all these things we regard as natural and we look forward to each in turn, but death is regarded as unnatural and is feared. When a woman conceives she spends nine long dreaming months thinking about and planning for her baby, but the thought that her birth gift to the child is inevitable death is something that never crosses her mind. Even if it did, she would not give up the joy of giving birth to what she has conceived. Men, even as children, know instinctively that their mother is also the primal cause of their death, and see her as the Nightmare of their childish dreams. Yet deep within every woman there is an instinctive knowledge concerning death: she knows, somewhere, somehow, that death is an illusion, and has the inner faith to bring her children into the world to face the inevitable journey into the unknown. This faith is the power of death on the first level.

Every pregnancy carries a risk, even in this age of enlightened medicine. In past eras every birth was a journey to the gates of possible death for a woman. Yet it was a journey she made time and again with courage and love to bring back a new life in her arms. Once that life was established, it was cherished with a lion-like ferocity that men have come to know very well over the centuries, sometimes to their cost. There is in nearly every woman a determination to guard the life that she has brought to birth, even at the risk of her own. Faced with a choice of who to save and who to let die when husband and son are both drowning, the mother will save the child every time. However there have also been mothers who, with equal courage, have helped a beloved but pain-racked child to a final peace. This ability to make a choice is the power of death on the second level.

To have power, a *sacrificial* death must be a willing death on the part of the victim. This is why the death of Jesus of Nazareth held so much power and one of the reasons why his agony in the garden of Gethsemene was so poignant. But it always takes two to make the sacrifice – the one who gives the life and the one who stands back and allows it to happen – *because it must happen.* For Mary to have accepted that her son was to become a willing sacrifice she had to have been touched by the same divinity as his own. The courage of the mother standing by as her child dies for an ideal is the culmination of her power of death. It happens every day in this modern world where young soldiers are torn apart by bombs, where young men and women are taken as hostages and disappear without trace and where sons and husbands place their lives on the line every day, and there is almost always a mother, wife, sister or lover who lives with the day-to-day knowledge that he may not return. To watch a beloved son, or even several sons march off to a war they did not start, and to let them go with grace, this is power. Deep in their racial mind men understand this, that their women will let them go, will mourn them if they do not return and will offer their power to them as they die if death is their destiny. This is the power of death on the third level.

A woman's power can be offered to a man if the woman is willing. If she is foolish he can take her power from her, sometimes without her noticing for a long time. Ideally the power is loaned for a time and then given back with love. Power is offered between lovers, given and received, and returned. In love there should be no losers and no victors, only those who share. A woman offers her body, opening the sacred temple of herself to a welcome guest. A man enters, bearing the gift of his seed, but he remains a guest, he does not own the temple.

# The Dying God

If woman, as the earthly image of the Great Mother Goddess, is a symbol of the eternal and limitless outpouring of spiritual life, then man, as the Sacrificed God, symbolizes the seasonal, fluctuating and limited side of earthly life. In the sexual cycle the woman is continually receptive to the male, but he is easily depleted and must rest before continuing the sexual union. In all cycle myths a God dies and goes down into the earth then a Goddess seeks him out and revitalizes him. In Her action of going down and into darkness, i.e. the womb, we see that the Goddess goes into Her own being and brings out, or gives birth to, the new God. This is the bottom line of the sacrifice myth: the Goddess conceives by the God, offers him as a sacrifice to the earth, then descends into Her own inner being to gestate his seed into the new God who, as Her son/consort, will impregnate Her and die in his turn. It is also the pattern of initiation, meaning 'rebirth', and is told in the stories of Jonah and the Whale, and the Raising of Lazarus, and of initiates lying for three days and nights in a sarcophagus before being taken up into a new life. It is also part of the underlying

love/hate relationship between mother and son and probably the
cause of the detestation throughout Western society of the sin of
incest.

# The Importance of the Phallus as a Male Symbol

In the funeral service of the Church of England the minister says,
'Man that is born of a woman hath but a short time to live . . . He
cometh up and is cut down like a flower.' This exactly describes
the cyclic power in a man. A man's power lies in his phallus, just
as a woman's power lies in her vulva (in the sense that it is the
seat of creative power), and the male erection is short-lived and
then 'cut down like a flower' – however, it does rise again. Male
pride has always been wrapped up in the symbol of the penis, and
men will go to great lengths to protect it and that which they
(mistakenly) think belongs to it, hence the invention of the chastity
belt. Ask any man what part of his anatomy he would least like to
part with and it is ten to one that the penis will be it. Cricket
'boxes', jock straps, boxing protectors, etc, are as much a part of a
sporting man's wardrobe as his suits and shirts. Watch a wall of
footballers lined up in front of the goal when a free kick is in the
offing. They could get their eyes damaged, their teeth knocked
out or their noses broken, but what do they clutch so protectively?
That's right.

The erect penis is an age-old symbol of manhood and power,
which is why kings and conquerors in ancient battles castrated
their male captives. It was a crude but effective means of ensuring
that as few as possible were going to bother them in the future. A
deposed king, such as Osiris, and any sons he might have were
also castrated to make certain that no one would be making a
claim to the throne. This was the reason for the flight of Isis and
Anubis from the vengeance of Set. Anubis, as the son of his father,
had to be kept from the same fate. It was the custom throughout
the known world at the time that a king *must* be whole and virile.
Anything less and the land and its people would suffer. This, as
you will recall, goes back to the linking of the land's fertility with
that of the king.

No matter how you may look at it in today's world, that symbol
of phallic power and strength remains deeply imbedded in the
racial subconscious. Because a woman, queen or priestess was
needed to prove that virility, anything and everything that drew

the female's attention to it was tried. The medieval short surcoat that ended just below the navel, worn with long hose and a bejewelled and probably padded codpiece, is a good example. Tight, well-worn and contour-hugging jeans with the zip casually lowered just enough to be suggestive are the modern equivalent, as the presenter of a British historical series found out. The series was one of the most popular of that year and women watched it in their thousands, *not* to see the stunning scenery or listen to the well-written commentary, but to watch the (admittedly good-looking) presenter in his well-worn jeans clambering about Greek mountains – though to be fair the poor man was truly wrapped up in his work and had little idea of the effect he was having on the female population of Great Britain!

The extended car bonnet, preferably with an unusual mascot, a powerful motor boat, a Kawasaki motor bike bristling with 'gadgets' or the time-honoured prancing stallion are all sexual euphemisms for the driver/rider's erect phallus. All are a part of the sexual display that every male animal hopes will win him a mate. The trouble is that the modern human female is far more likely to be turned on by a man's mind than his body!

# The Power of Man

## The Four Powers of Man

Man has four kinds of power, the four and the three together making the sacred number of seven. Woman is the creative triangle to the manifesting square of man. They were always designed to be interrelated.

The powers of man are as follows: strength, change, order and acceptance. Sometimes a man will try to adapt a woman's power for his own use, but it will never be completely successful, for no matter what type of man he is, he will always be the 'straight rod of direction' to her 'circle of containment'. Rather he must seek to adapt his own powers to match the kind he seeks. In this way he will strengthen his power.

### The Power of Strength
Physical strength has always been desirable in the male animal. In the herd animal where strength is used in the rutting season to gain a group of females, it meant the strongest and the best genes were passed on. This applied to early tribes as well and meant security for the species. In prehistoric times the human race endured cold, hunger and a hostile environment, so only the

strongest survived. But strength as a power had other uses, the most important of which to primitive man was the ability to conquer. To the strongest went the best land, the most fertile women and the greater share of food. As time went on he used his power to conquer other things: whole lands, races, and anyone who stood in his way. Then came the challenges of weaponry, science, disease, communication and transportation, and finally man conquered flight and went on into space. Strength to conquer used in the right way is the power of strength on the first level.

But strength of mind and will is equally important and the human male has also excelled at this form of strength throughout history. It is the determination to persevere, to so concentrate the mind that even when the body is useless it is forced to do what must be done, that is strength of mind. Making a stand against something twice your size is mental strength, yet Stone Age man did it every day. It took strength of mind to stand in the way of a wounded bison with only a stone spear in your hand, but if it had not been there in the heart and sinew of the prehistoric hunters, we as a species would not have made it to the Bronze Age.

Strength of will also would have been needed to open the mind to new things and extend thinking, to invent, refine and teach. Out of this strength came writing, language, and the ability to discuss and argue. As his mind began to explore not only the outer world but also the inner world, man would have discovered the primal nightmare: that within his head, he was alone. Yet time and again men have bent their will to the task of making sense of the world around them. To bend the will to a task and master it, that is the power of strength on the second level.

Who first thought about thought itself, or wondered about the beginning of the world? When did man first begin to 'imagine' and use imagination to cause changes to happen? Who gave a woman the first real kiss? Who first made an offering to that *Something* he could not understand? Whoever he was, he was showing a spiritual strength. Man, for all his blunderings, has always felt the presence of a Creator and been able to trust that the body held something more than a moment of life, that there was something beyond the darkness of death. The early thinkers like Thales, Anaximander and Anaximenes were the first to observe and use the abstract mind to think in three dimensions and they had the courage to teach this skill to others. This is the power of strength on the third level.

*The Power of Change*
The power of change on the physical level stems from the natural curiosity of the human animal. It is the need to expand into a new environment, a new tribe, a new way of life. It is the power that

took life out of the oceans and onto dry land, made it come out of the trees into the savannah. It was this power that made man the species stand upright and make the first tool. Later on the desire for change turned him from a nomadic hunter into a farmer and domesticator of the wild sheep and oxen. It was man's power to change things that brought the wild dog into his house as a guardian and friend, a house that was itself a change from the early cave. The human male has always needed, even craved for change, and it spurred him on to invent the wheel that gave him freedom to wander from place to place or to carry ever increasing yields from field to market. Change, once implemented, never stops and man goes on changing himself, his way of life, his planet, and in time, the universe. This is the power of change on the first level.

Always there have been men different from the others, men with a far-off look in the eyes, with eyes that saw things differently. They seemed more than human . . . or less than human. They were men who could change and become animals, birds and other, less inviting, things. The shape changers were the first shamans – and they still move among us. The power to change in the mind and make the change real is a gift that has its roots so far back in history that we cannot seek it out. Then there is the changing of history itself, the moment in time when the answer to a question will set in motion a change that will affect future events for hundreds, even thousands of years.

As the physical brain of mankind altered and grew, so did the uses to which that brain was put. Abstract thought, once established, brought about things like conscience, ethics and empathy with other human beings and of course the magical influence of music and musical notation. This change was not always comfortable – sometimes it was downright dangerous – but it went on growing. Concepts of education, learning, art and drama made their appearance, the latter growing out of temple rituals. Perception was a big part of this change within the actual brain. Colour vision became more acute as the practice of art became more widespread and man needed to see and use more subtle shades. The changes within and around man became faster and faster, feeding his mental desire to seek new information. The ability to change mental patterns and use them to stimulate further changes is the power of change on the second level.

Yet the practice of those beliefs came slowly. For thousands of years the Mother had ruled over the spirituality of humankind. Then began the slow changeover to the rule of the Father God. The old ways of worship drew to a close and monotheism gradually took over from the pantheons of the old world. Religious change brought about questions, and among them were the twin

questions about sex and sin. Man questioned many things at this
time about God and God's plan for the world and for humanity.
He also began to make comparisons between himself and God and
for the first time the primal divinity of men and women was
spoken about openly. These discussions and arguments were to
go on for over 2,000 years. There are still changes to face, for once
you become aware of change you see it everywhere. The ability to
accept that religion, like everything else, must change is the power
of change on the third level.

*The Power of Order*
The first set of man-made laws that really had any effect must
have been the Code of Hammurabi. This remarkable king ruled
Babylon in approximately 1700 BC. His code was noted for its
justice and fairness, especially to women, for no other set of laws
either before that time or in the later medieval times gave women
so much say in their own affairs. From this time man set about
creating order at all levels of physical life. Criminal law, social law,
religious law, all were part of the new order of things and were
implemented with a sometimes heavy hand. Jewish law was the
harshest and its punishments were often death, usually by stoning
or by the sword. But men also began to see law and order in the
natural world about them, and the very beginnings of the law of
physics were emerging. Experiments and observation yielded the
information that although man might impinge his laws on people,
there were far greater and vaster laws that moved in unison with
the cosmos. The ability to see order in the natural law of the
universe is the power of order on the first level.

Education gives order and accessibility to knowledge and stores
it in the mind. Therefore education is rightly one of the main
concerns of the modern world, though in earlier times learning
was confined to the nobility and to the Church. With the event of
the Renaissance, man set his mind to the acquiring of knowledge
and also to its storage for the future. Caxton's invention of the
printing press enabled man for the first time to make many copies
of the same book – unfortunately it also spelt the demise of the
trained memory and the ancient 'mouth to ear' way of teaching.
There is a price for everything.

Another part of the power of order is the practice of logic, and
this discipline has played a large part in man's thinking processes
from the early philosophers onwards. This is not to say that logic
can seem to be sadly absent at times! Nevertheless education,
literature and the precision of mind and thought is the power of
order on the second level.

The ability to perceive and recognize the beauty of order in
spiritual regions has resulted in some of our most wonderful

descriptive prose, and the mystic has played a large part in the history of man and religion, stemming mostly from the time of the changeover from the worship of the Mother to that of the Father. It has always been difficult to translate into words the glory of what is seen on the higher levels, and for the most part the symbolic language chosen is that of human love, love being the highest and best emotion in humankind. The love poems of St John of the Cross remain unsurpassed in their ability to show us the spiritual order of the cosmos. The recognition of that higher order and the ability to contact it, even briefly, is the power of order on the third level.

## The Power of Acceptance

To accept things is not always easy, in fact acceptance is sometimes the hardest thing we ever have to do. On the earth level man has had to accept that he is restricted by his very humanity. Though he came from the sea, he can only return to it by using his inventiveness and ingenuity to help him breathe. He can fly, but only by using his mind to construct machines to help him. He can only run so fast, live so long, climb so high, endure so much pain. He is finite, he is limited, he must accept that he can only do so much. . . . He must also accept that he will always *try* to go one better. To know one's limits and accept them, and then still try to exceed them, that is the power of acceptance on the first level.

Another thing that may be hard to accept is that within the mind we are all, each and every one of us, totally and utterly alone.[1] We can share most of our thoughts and ideas, we can become so close to certain people it seems as if they are a mental part of us, but it is an illusion and one we must accept. A lifetime is spent in gathering knowledge and experience, and most of it we can pass on to others, teaching them with love and care, but the finer points, the indefinable instinct that makes us unique, that cannot be passed on. It will go with us into the infinite and be gathered into that part of ourselves that endures from incarnation to incarnation. To accept this and not allow it to turn us from our path of gathering experience, this is the power of acceptance on the second level.

In the early mystery religions the most important advice given to the neophyte was: 'Know thyself.' This is without doubt one of the most difficult things for anyone to do. What is even more difficult is to accept yourself, as you are, at this moment, knowing all the worst of yourself and all the best of yourself, the failures

---

[1] However there is reason to believe that this solipsistic universe of the self borders on another mental universe common to us all. This is a phenomenon just beginning to be explored by magicians.

and the successes, the hopes, fears, dreams and nightmares. To know exactly where you are on the ladder of evolution and to accept it, that is to be in balance with the universe, even if there is a long way yet to go. To know this, to accept this, is to know the power of acceptance on the third level.

Because I have assigned various powers to male and female does not mean that only that sex has access to those powers. Both sexes have a part and a share in all the powers. I have known men with a very vital power of life and women who had all three levels of the powers of order at their fingertips. Everyone has a portion of every power, but in varying degrees. What I am saying is that each sex specializes in certain powers and these are, in general, better suited to its use. A woman excels in those pertaining to birth, life, and death because they are her ancient powers and are still in her keeping. But the powers of men are as ancient and as vital. Instead of trying to move in on each other's powers it would be better for the world and the New Age if they were used to support each other.

The Lords of the Dark Face will always take advantage of our human weaknesses and one of those weaknesses is the jealousy that still exists between some types of men and women. The answer is *love*, for love is the foundation of balance and harmony, and one of the major expressions of love is a sexual relationship with a bonded partner. It is not the only way to express love, but it is the way described and offered in this book. I repeat, love is the foundation.

# 3. THE VIEWPOINT OF THE CHURCH

Women and sex have been the two targets of the Christian Church for centuries. In early times, especially in Hellenic Greece, women had certain rights. They were allowed to divorce a cruel husband, or one who became mad or violent. They had their ways of contraception and it was seen as their right to use it. They could own property and even administer it in some areas. In short, they were considered to be the rightful 'other half' of humanity.

By contrast the Church, right down through the ages, has persistently railed against woman, calling her evil, debased and the originator of sin. Most of this is due to St Paul's incessant hostility to the female sex. He may well have written some of the most quoted parts of the Bible, and he may well have brought Christianity to the rest of the world, but he remains an embittered personality who caused much suffering to women. His attitude towards sex was just as bad, his rejection of the gift given to man by the Creator prompting Cerinthus to say, 'Man should not be ashamed of what God has not been ashamed to create.'

Contrast this with the following (and I quote from Charles Seltman's invaluable book *Women in Antiquity*):

> The [so-called] secluded and despised Athenian women ran homes, bullied their husbands with no fear of them, ran wild at festivals, went to the theatre, took lovers, drank wine . . . the landowning women of Sparta . . . the young matrons of Lydia and Tuscany famed for their beauty and light hearted promiscuity . . . the Hetairai . . . enjoying the freedom of the woman unattached . . .

There is no doubt who got the best deal. As far as Paul and the early Church Fathers were concerned (by the way, where were the early Church Mothers?) sex was something that kept man's mind away from God. This I find hard to believe, when anyone who has ever been in love and made love will tell you that sex brings you closer to the divine than at any other time.

Paul took the biblical story of Adam and Eve to be absolute truth and therefore believed with fervour in blaming the woman. However if we read the Bible we see that when God came rampaging through the Garden of Eden heaven bent on finding out who had been 'scrumping'[1] His apples, He found Adam holding the 'core' of the disturbance in his hand. On being asked about this damning piece of evidence, Adam, ever the gentleman, pointed to Eve and said, 'She made me do it . . .' or words to that effect.

This was the first buck-passing in pseudo-history, and that is all the Bible is. Not a word of it can be *proven* as actual truth. It is a collection of myth, legends, allegorical tales and writings put down, in some cases, centuries after the event, then mistranslated and twisted out of sight to suit the purpose of what was at the time a minor religious sect.

When we look back over the past, we see repressed men, sadistic popes and a cruel priesthood that on the one hand denounced, and rightly so, the cruel child sacrifices of Moloch, but on the other racked, tortured and burnt women, children and babies (some born to women in the process of being burnt and tossed back on to the flames)[2] for no crime other than malicious gossip, the fact that they were old and lived alone with a cat for company, had property the Church wanted, or held a different belief – even if it was a Christian belief like that of the Cathars – from their own. The Protestants hated the Catholics, the Catholics hated the Pagans, Luther hated the Jews, Calvin hated everything . . . and they all slaughtered each other every chance they got.

This is a Church founded on love, preached by a wise and gentle man who had recognized his own divinity and relationship to the Creator and wanted to share it with everyone, not just Jews. He *was* a Jew, by the way, he lived and died a Jew and would probably have been horrified to be thought of as anything else. He attended weddings and drank the health of the bride and groom, he healed the sick, no matter whether they were Roman and worshipped their own Gods, or whether they were Jews. He even took pity on the demons and allowed them to withdraw from their 'host' and take refuge in a herd of swine. Yeshua of Nazareth cannot be blamed for what has been done in his name, and he was got rid of for similar reasons, for worshipping in a different way from those around him.

The early Christians were almost morbidly fixed on celibacy and virginity. Tales are told of young girls, vulnerable at the age of puberty because of their feminine link with the inner levels, who allowed themselves to be put to death, usually in the most painful

---

[1] An English idiom meaning 'to steal'.
[2] This fact has been recorded in accounts of witch trials.

and sexually debauched of ways. Breasts were torn off with hot irons, red-hot swords were thrust into the vagina and/or anus – and all because they had been brainwashed into believing that their virginity, if preserved, assured them of a place in heaven. Books about such martyrs were considered educational reading for young Victorian children, and we worry about television violence today! This kind of influence over young minds shows how sick some fanatics can get.

However, as any psychologist will tell you, sex, when repressed, will come out in other ways. It is after all the most powerful of all human urges, linked to the most powerful of all, the urge to survive, because it offers a way for the species to survive as against personal survival. It has been rightly said that what you fear, you become: hide sex away and it will emerge in a different form, usually in art, as that which is creative will always find a creative outlet. We find it doing just that in medieval paintings of the Virgin and in those of Jesus on the Cross with the wound in his side looking suspiciously like the female labia, from which, having been pierced by the phallic spear, gushes a mixture of blood and water as the Christ is born into a higher world. We see voyeurism depicted in paintings such as 'Susanna and the Elders', 'Esther and the King', and of course 'Eve and the Serpent'. I remember my late mother-in-law being highly embarrassed at seeing a painting in the museum at Monserrat in northern Spain depicting an elderly Hebrew prophet being breast fed by his daughter who was visiting him in jail. (His captors were trying to starve him to death.) There is a painting extant of St Bernard of Clairvaux being fed by the Virgin Mary from her breast as a mark of favour. The cult of the mother is a cult also of her womanhood and femininity, her breasts and her vulva, those organs which make her a woman. Misogynists have mothers even if they despise them!

Has the Church changed its views on women? Not a lot. Women are still barred by their sex from reclaiming the ancient title of 'priestess', for example. (If we ever do get it back, are we going to let them style us as 'women priests'? I hope not. Let us make a stand to win back the older and rightful title, which is so much more suitable – and perhaps we can come up with something more feminine than a cassock!)

Celibacy is still demanded of its priests by the Catholic Church though there are rebels within the Church who are trying to change this. Should being a priest deny a man the fire and beauty of a sexual relationship? It might just make him more sympathetic to his flock and to women in particular.

Contraception was practised in the old world, but in ours, with far more dependable ways of doing it, more than half the world is denied its use, not on medical grounds, or even because of non-availability, but because the Church of Rome says it is wrong. This is based on the 'be fruitful and multiply' edict of the Bible, given in an era when the total population of the known world was probably less than that of modern London. Never mind that we are running out of clean air, natural resources, water, land, food and those species that share the planet with us. Never mind that in Latin America women are dying at 30, worn out with continual childbirth in dangerous and medically unsafe conditions. Sex, which should be a wonderful and uplifting experience between two people, is becoming an opiate against despair and poverty, lessening its glory and its godliness.

# Sex and the Bible

O that you would kiss me with the kisses of your mouth!
For your love is better than wine
– *The Song of Solomon 1:2.*

Show me a choirboy who has not looked up the sexy bits in the Bible! There is plenty of sex to find there, not least in the Song of Solomon, some lines of which are quoted above, and in the laws pertaining to marriage, in particular the Law of Leverite Marriage. This states that if a woman was left a widow and had no children, her husband's nearest male relative was required by law to take her as a wife and raise up children to her dead husband that 'his name be not blotted out of Israel'. If that nearest relative declined then, in the words of the Deuteronomic Code, the wife in the presence of witnesses would go up to him, pull off his sandal and spit in his face. This idea of taking in a dead relative's wife is a very old one and it provided the woman with a home and a family of her own. The story of Ruth and Boaz is a good example of this law, even down to the taking off of the sandal by he who declined to take Ruth to wife and gave her instead to Boaz. In passing it is interesting to note that such gatherings of elders to act as witnesses and pass judgements were always held by the *gates* of the city where the two pillars or pylons that formed the entrance acted as the *pillars of the temple* or *scales of justice* – a faint memory of a past age, the Age of Gemini and the Twin Pillars.

Polygamy was practised widely in biblical times, as it still is in the Middle East. Many of the patriarchs of the Old Testament had more than one wife, Abraham being one of them. In addition to Sarah there was also Keturah, who bore him several children, and his concubine Hagar the Egyptian, who bore to him Ishmael, the ancestor of the Arab race. As all this was accomplished, so we are told, when Abraham was well over 80 years old, and as he went on to sire children at the age of 100, it does seem that, like Moses, his 'natural force was not abated' with age.

The men of the old world seem to have been a sprightly lot. David had eight wives and numerous concubines, but his son Solomon topped them all for it is said that he had over a thousand wives. But it was to Balkis, Queen of Sheba, sometimes called 'the Queen of the South', that he gave his greatest love. She came to him on a state visit, having heard of his great wisdom, and captivated him with her beauty and her ability to match him in knowledge. She refused at first to mate with him, but he resorted to trickery and to keep her promise she yielded. When read in its entirety and with background knowledge, however, the story is one of a ritual marriage with a highly-powered intention. Let us not forget that Solomon was a master magician. The intention was the conception of Menelek, traditionally called the Ethiopian Master.

Legend abounds too with stories of the Ring of Solomon. The Hidden Tradition says that it was sent to Balkis on the birth of her son, and that it remains hidden in the land of Ethiopia awaiting the one destined to find it. Menelek is the Winged Lion, one of the Four Hidden Masters of the World. All of these Masters were ritually conceived in the beginning by what was once called the Rite of Nuit, or the Rite of Hat-Hor, but which is now simply the Great Rite.

If we look now at the story of Esther we can trace through the convoluted theme a very clear picture of a ritual surviving from the earliest times: the testing of the virility of the king. Much is made of the number *seven*, the traditional number of years after which the reigning king had to prove his manhood. The king in question here is Ahasuerus and we are told that he feasted *seven* important men for *seven* days. On the seventh day he sent his *seven* chamberlains to his queen to tell her to come before him. She refused. Maybe she did not relish the thought of being taken sexually before the whole court just to prove that the king was still virile. For this she was deposed for having disregarded the law.

To replace her they gathered together all the young virgins of the land. (Ahasuerus's rule extended from India to Ethiopia.) Among them was Esther, a young girl who had been brought up in Babylon by her uncle when the Jews had been taken into exile by Nebuchadnezzar. This gives us the clue we are looking for, for in Babylon this custom of testing the king was well known – which makes Esther the ideal queen/priestess for Ahasuerus.

The Bible makes a point of telling us not once but three times that there were given to the virgins 'their things for purification'. Clearly this is working up to what we can only believe is an important ritual. Esther was also given *seven* maidens for her servants. Her obvious knowledge of what was required of her made her a favourite with Hegai, the powerful eunuch keeper of the women's quarters, so it is hardly surprising that she was the one on whom the king's choice fell.

Things went well until the Jews of the city and the provinces were accused of disloyalty to the king and the order went out to destroy them. Esther, in order to plead for them and to accuse those who would destroy her people, went before the king without being sent for, *something punishable by death unless the king offered mercy by holding out his golden sceptre to be touched.*

The exact words are: '. . . and the king held out to Esther the golden sceptre that was in his hand. So Esther drew near and touched the top of the sceptre.' Knowing what we do, we can safely assume that what she touched was the phallus of the king, for in offering this vital part of his body for her to touch, he was giving her his trust. On the next day Esther again came with a petition for the king and he granted it, whereupon the ringleader of the would-be usurpers tried to rape her in her bed. Understandably the king hanged him. Due to Esther's efforts on their behalf, the Jews regained their freedom and property and were given permission to seek out their enemies and slay them. Out of these days came the Feast of Purim.

The act of public sex was fairly common in most parts of the Middle East at this time. Usually it was the celebration of a particular ritual, or to make a point, for example the fitness of the king, or to make a claim on the kingship. This was the reason why Absalom, the son of David, in order to claim his father's kingdom and (what was more important) to be *seen* to do it, spread a tent on the top of David's house and, in the language of the Bible, 'went in unto his father's concubines in the sight of all Israel' (2 Samuel 16:22).

There are many more instances in the Bible to indicate sexual rites, and non-Jewish temples complete with priests and priestesses were fairly commonplace in Palestine. Jezebel, the queen who was so despised, is quite clearly the priestess of an ancient tradition, and suffers a ritualistic death at the hands of the mob for that reason. To do justice to such a wide subject would mean a lengthy research of the synoptic gospels, comparing one to the other, but there is no doubt that it would yield results.

# Adam and Eve and Lilith

This biblical *ménage à trois* has been the source of more books, paintings and speculation than anything else in the Bible. There are those who take it – and indeed everything else in the Bible – quite literally, but most see it for what it is: a rather disjointed allegory. The eating of the Apple of Knowledge could well be a race memory of the time in our history when men were ignorant of their part in conception, and the women saw to it that they stayed that way.

As we have already seen, Adam was not keen on taking his share of blame. Having been forbidden to eat of the Tree of Knowledge, he did just that, not understanding that sometimes initiates are told not to do things in order to see if they will make up their own minds. Eve was the one with an understanding of what the Fruit of Knowledge might entail and the courage to taste it. To dare, to will, to know and to keep silent: these are the virtues of the initiate.

Adam's behaviour did not improve once they were established on earth, having been clothed with 'garments of skin' by their Creator. Legend tells us that the serpent followed them to Earth and, in his original form of a Son of the Morning, lay with Eve and got her with child (the phallic symbolism of the serpent here is obvious). Some say that Cain was the son of the serpent and not of Adam. Abel, however, was his son. Although the Jews had a long list of laws forbidding marriage within certain family limits, the Old Testament is full of contradictions. We are told of the birth of Cain and Abel and that when they grew up they had wives . . . but if Adam and Eve were the first and only couple, where did the wives come from if they were not the daughters of that same couple?

After the death of Abel at the hand of his brother Adam left the bed of Eve and wandered about the Earth for 130 years – which would have been taking abstinence to the extreme if he had not met up with Lilith once more.

Lilith is without doubt one of the most fascinating characters in the Bible. The first wife of Adam, she left him because he insisted on the topmost position during sex. It might well be that this story came out of the changeover from the worship of the female to that of the male – it has that sort of feel to it. Lilith, along with the Goddess Isis (and the camel) was the holder of the secret name of God, and this gave her a great deal of power. After rejecting Adam's demands that she take the subordinate position in their lovemaking, she leapt up, pronouncing the Name of God, and 'forthwith she grew wings and flew away'.

The men stuck together as usual and Adam complained to God, saying, 'The woman thou gavest to me has left me.' God promptly sent three angels after her to bring her back to Adam. Quite rightly she refused, and for this she was cursed to bring forth hundreds of children each day, of which one hundred would die before nightfall. Only the male mind could think up such a cruel punishment for a woman!

God had apparently found it much more difficult to make a woman than a man. (That figures.) He made several attempts, three in fact, before finally coming up with Eve. The first time he allowed Adam to watch as he made her, a process which so revolted Adam that he declined the finished product! The second version was no better, but finally Eve was created, and God plaited her hair, adorned her like a bride with 24 pieces of jewellery and presented her to Adam . . . who was entranced.*

It is obvious that Eve and Lilith are really two sides to the same woman. This division is still a part of female psychology: the practical, womanly, motherly Eve, and the fiery, unpredictable, sexual temptress Lilith. Both have courage to defy God, something Adam would never have done. For this both have been reviled down the ages: Eve, as the cause of the Fall of Adam, is condemned to bear her children in pain and anguish; Lilith is to be looked on as the killer of children, although this last is contradicted for she is also the Goddess who plays with children while they sleep, causing them to dream and smile.†

This subject is so wide it is impossible to cover it adequately in this book, so I propose to continue and extend coverage in a future book, *Daughters of Eve*, which in many ways will be a second volume to this one. For those who cannot wait to find out I recommend Ean Begg's *The Cult of the Black Virgin* and Barbara Black Koltuv's *The Book of Lilith*.

* R. Graves and R. Patai, *Hebrew Myths: The Book of Genesis*, McGraw-Hill, New York, 1963.
† R. Patai, *The Hebrew Goddess*, Ktav Publishing House, Hoboken, 1967, and *The Gates to the Old City*, Avon, New York, 1980.

# 4. THE FORBIDDEN ASPECTS OF SEX

What is acceptable and lawful in one area of the world is damned in another. As Kipling has written, '. . . the wildest dreams of Kew are facts in Katmandu, and the crimes of Clapham chaste in Martaban.' How you think and act is conditioned by where and how you live. Where the act of sex is concerned, it appears that almost everything, at some time or another, has been either condoned or banned.

East and West have very opposite views and sex is certainly one area where it is very hard for 'the twain to meet'. The East has rarely had any difficulty in accepting sexuality and its place in both social and religious life. The West, on the other hand, has always had the greatest difficulty in giving it a place in either of those areas. One of the greatest of our Western taboos is that of incest, yet it has always been there, to our shame, and if we believe what the media tell us, it is even on the increase. In isolated country areas it was almost a part of life a few centuries ago. A farmer with two or three daughters and a dead wife would think little of using one of the daughters as a substitute wife. Child abuse was rife in Victorian times, when a prostitute might be as young as eight or nine. In India a child bride of the same age even today is not rare, although the husband will, at least in most cases, wait until his bride is sexually mature before consummating the marriage. There are some states in America where marriage is legal when the girl is 13.

Political marriages in the past have been made when the children were barely out of the cradle – girls of three and four married to men older than their fathers, boys married to women much older. There is on record a letter from a queen to her daughter, already married at the age of 11 to an older man and a thousand miles from her family, telling her to 'hurry up and become a woman, as it is of the utmost importance that [you bear] a son as soon as possible'. Small wonder that women died so early and so quickly in childbirth.

In Ancient Egypt, however, it was considered quite normal for both sexes to marry as soon as puberty was reached. In the royal houses, father married daughter (Akenaten married several of his), brother married sister, and mother married son. In this way the bloodline was kept pure, a purity that soon backfired when inbreeding brought about congenital deformations and increased the chances of hereditary disease. Often this intermarriage was bound up with the need for the male to be enroyalled by the female, something we have discussed earlier. Even today there are isolated places in North America where inter-family breeding is almost a way of life.

Incest between father and daughter is found even in the Bible (Genesis 19:30–8). Lot, the nephew of Abraham, went up into the hills with his two daughters and dwelt there in a cave. Both girls were unmarried and desired children so they plotted to make their father drunk and each girl in turn spent a night with him. This resulted in the birth of Moab, ancestor of the Moabites, and Ben-Ammi, ancestor of the Ammonites.

When Amnon, the son of King David, raped his half-sister she begged him not to break the law, but first to speak to the king for, she said, 'He will not withhold me from you' – which would appear to be saying that had he asked first, his father would indeed have given him his half-sister in marriage, even against the law.

Anal intercourse between man and wife is still a forbidden act in many places – which is not to say it does not take place. One of the accusations flung against the Cathars was that they 'used their wives *per anum*', and this, along with further accusations of bestiality and buggery, from a king and a pope who were probably into similar practices! If they were they would not have been the first to indulge. The legends that surround the persona of Richard the Lionheart of England never go into the fact that he was more than once required by the Church to pay fines for the 'sin of sodomy' – fines that in today's money would amount to something like a quarter of a million pounds.

It is only within the last quarter of a century that the law concerning homosexuality between consenting adults has been repealed, although there are areas where that law still holds, at least for the moment. But by and large the whole area of homosexuality and gay love is now an openly accepted lifestyle with magazines, books, clubs, and stores that cater for homosexuals, without prejudice. It is no longer a source of gossip when two women or two men set up house together, although in earlier times it would have meant the stake, for not only witches were burnt. The abusive term 'faggot' for a homosexual stems from the practice of binding them round with straw and placing them around the stake. These unfortunates were literally used as faggots to start the pyre.

# The Danger in Indiscriminate Use

Although I have sung the praises of sex as a sensual pleasure and as a means of worship, no one but a fool would pretend that there are no dangers in its use.

There is a popular idea still held in many areas that syphilis came back with the returning crusaders. However, of late there have been other speculations that it arrived in Europe from Haiti, brought back to Portugal by those sailors who had gone to the New World with Columbus. There is a great deal of controversy about this and personally I doubt it will ever be fully decided. What matters is that it *did* arrive and spread with unbelievable rapidity throughout the rest of Europe and beyond.

In his book *Sex in History*, G. Rattray Taylor states that 'it reached France, Germany, and Switzerland in 1485, Scotland in 1497, Hungary and Russia in 1499. It got to India in 1498 and China in 1505.' (In 1506 the Archbishop of Crete died of it!)

Today we have an even more deadly disease in the form of AIDS. Strangely enough, there are reports that this disease also came from Haiti. Like syphilis, no one can be sure of its origin, only its deadly effect on all who contract it. In a similar fashion to rabies, once it has taken hold nothing can stop its inevitable ending.

Because of these things the rituals in this book *must* be kept for those who are in a steady and stable relationship. I cannot emphasize this too strongly. To go into any kind of ritual untrained and unprepared is wrong, dangerous and misguided. To go into a series of sexually-orientated rituals with someone you do not know well is the height of foolishness. The use of condoms is advised not simply as a precaution against unwanted pregnancy but as a safeguard for both partners, especially where they are magical partners only and not bonded, whether the bond be a legal one or a handfasting.

Syphilis and AIDS are only two of many kinds of infection that can be contracted or passed sexually. Gonorrhoea and herpes are also on the list. The rule has to be: if in doubt, don't. You owe it to your partner and yourself to be clean and free from any kind of infection. Apart from which, anything offered to the Gods should be pure and clean and the best you have to give.

# Morals and Ethics

We all have personal standards that we keep to and which we will not allow ourselves to go beyond. There are a few people who do not, and the Gods deal with such in their own ways. There will always be those who elect themselves as the guardians of other people's morals – mostly they are themselves disturbed, afraid, and a prey to their own dark inner fears. They use the power they gain over others as substitute for other, more natural, energies. It always amazes me how such people know about certain articles in certain magazines, or which film is (in their opinion) objectionable, or who is doing what with whom and when. They must go out of their way to find out, to pry, to slide in and out of bookshops carrying armfuls of soft porn magazines!

Films are always a safe bet. Some people found *The Life of Brian* objectionable. Fine, let them switch it off, they do not have to see it – but neither should they have the power to tell me I cannot see it. I loved it; I found it funny, moving, and very apt. It made the story real for the first time, showing us what it would have been like to wake up one morning to find yourself hailed as the Messiah.

Nudity in films and on stage is sometimes an integral part of the life the piece is trying to portray. It is only a couple of decades since the Hollywood censor never allowed a double bed in a scene, just twin beds with a table – usually a large one – between them. Again, if nudity offends you, you do not have to see it.

The usual grouse is that young people will be led astray by such things. Rubbish, young people are led astray by drunken violent and abusive fathers, drug pushers outside their schools, mothers who leave them to roam the streets late at night while they play bingo. They are led astray by shopkeepers who sell them alcohol, cigarettes, or glue for sniffing, and who allow cards advertising the sale of sex to be displayed in their windows. They are led astray by sheer boredom. More children are shocked and distressed by the sex films shown in school biology lessons than by anything on television. If you think they are frightened by violence on the small screen, ask any psychologist and they will tell you that a young child is one of the most naturally violent creatures around. Only when the violence is shown as victorious or as an admirable way of life does it cross the dividing line. Some of the most violent films are actually *made* for children – look at the transformation of the witch in *Snow White* for example, the fight between the prince and the witch in *Sleeping Beauty*, the prejudice in *Dumbo*, and maliciousness in *Cinderella*. Yet children thrive on such stories. They know whom to cheer and whom to boo. The inner censor is the one to obey: parents have the right to say 'no'. I have the right to put this book together: you have the right not to read it. My ethics demand that I tell those who pick it up in the store that this book can be dangerous if you are not trained. Those same ethics demand that I refuse to take into my school anyone I do not think is stable enough for the work, or who is under the age where he or she can make up their own mind safely.

Ethics also demand that my right to believe and worship in the way I have chosen without being persecuted is as unequivocal as that given to a Jew, a Hindu, a Muslim, or a Buddhist. Without such basic rights no man or woman is truly free.

To those who will buy and use this book I say: ethics are your guideline. In your use of these rituals make sure no one is harmed or betrayed. Behave towards your partner with gentleness and courtesy. Do not use the rituals as an excuse for other things.

Do not betray your own inner divinity.

# 5. SEX IN ANCIENT CULTURES AND IN MODERN TIMES

According to some of the early thinkers and philosophers the key to the mysteries of the universe lay hidden in the mysteries of sex. On the one hand there existed the fiery, active, male generative power and on the other the gentle, passive, receptive, female power. Out of these two powers all else was created. Most of what we would call the polytheistic religions also ran along these lines, their male Gods supplying the generative powers and the Goddesses the receptive. Occasionally there would be those that crossed over and the Fire Goddesses such as Vesta, Pele, Sekmet and Kali emerged, while to complement them there came about the less aggressive Gods such as Mercury the Messenger, Thoth the Scribe, and Aesculapius the Healer.

## The Ancient World

Sex pervaded every aspect of life in ancient times. It was considered an important part of humanity's existence. The genitals were not considered to be obscene and in some countries they were barely covered. The decorations on Greek pottery have left us with what amounts to a film show of what life was like. Much of it is highly sexual in content: satyrs and nymphs cavort naked under the olive trees, young men and women pass by, bathing, dancing and making love, drawn from life as the artists saw it happen. The Greeks fought their battles either naked or nearly so and saw nothing strange in it.

The Romans were less inclined to nudity but still had their festivals at which all pretence to modesty and shyness were abandoned. In fact their Bacchanalian festivals became so bad, so obscene and violent, that finally they were banned.

Meanwhile in Egypt, under the fierce heat, the women wore

little more than a shift of transparent linen, while female slaves seldom wore anything more than beads and the men of the household wore a brief pleated kilt of the same material. A woollen cloak might be added at night if it grew chilly.

## Phoenicia

The Phoenicians called their chief God Asshur, or Asher, meaning the penis, the happy one (note the similarity to Eheieh Asher Eheieh, given as a name by Yaweh to Moses in his exile). Another of their Gods was Dagon. Represented as half-fish and half-man, he was a teacher of mankind who came up out of the sea each day and returned at night. The fish was worshipped as a fertility symbol because of the female fish's ability to lay many thousands of eggs and because it lived in the life-giving ocean. The practice of young women impaling themselves on the stone phallus of Asshur prior to their wedding night was commonplace.

## Egypt

The Land of the Pharoahs has drawn the imagination of everyone at some time or another. Its religion was complex in the extreme with many Gods. It breaks down roughly into two groups of deities, those headed by Ra and those headed by Osiris. The Osirian group is the one with which most people are familiar. To the Star Goddess Nuit and the Earth God Geb were born two sets of twins: Osiris and Isis, Nephthys and Set, one set with a light skin and the other dark.

Osiris and his sister/wife took human form as the king and queen of Khem, the ancient name of Egypt. Osiris was the symbol of the generative power of nature. In fact he was basically a corn God. To show his power to rise again after being cut down, he was sometimes depicted with three phalloi. The creation myth of the Egyptians speaks of Atum the Creator masturbating into his clenched fist, and there are many representations of Atum and other Gods in this position. Some carry rods or sceptres with a phallic head, others are shown with an erect penis, being adored by worshippers and anointed with oils and perfumes. Herodotus described a religious procession in which small statues with movable sex organs attached to a cord were carried to the temple.

The worship of the Apis bull was a part of the Egyptians' sacred rites and the French traveller Vivant Denon speaks of the finding of the embalmed phallus of a bull interred with a female mummy. Their rituals were, however, much more rigid and stylized than those of the exuberant Hellenes: they opted for dignity rather than excess.

# Greece

Zeus was the king of the Greek pantheon, and his origin can be traced from the Vedic *Dyaus pitar* or Ζευπατερ. He was a sky God and as such most of his 'amours' (and there were plenty) were with human women. (We can see an echo in this of the biblical story of the Sons of God and the Daughters of Men and their intermarriage.) The children that were born of these women were the demi-gods, the heroes who were deified after death. It is also of some significance that Zeus was called the Aegis-Bearer, as was his daughter Athena, who was born without a mother, from the head of Zeus. The aegis was a ritual goat pelt worn by a chieftain or ruler and was the totem of the Aegidae, a tribe that moved into Greece in its early history. The goat, like Zeus himself, was exceptionally prolific and this may have accounted for the aegis being part of his symbology. The worship of the goat as a giver of fertility was widespread over many lands and religions, extending from India in the north to the famous Temple of Mendes in the Nile Delta. Zeus was also given to what was styled even in ancient times as Greek love, i.e. homosexuality. His abduction of the beautiful Κουροσ or youth, Ganymede, in the form of an eagle has been the subject of many paintings.

Hermes was, like his father, much given to the pursuit of women and even his famous staff, the caduceus, depicted the male and female snakes twined about the upright staff or lingam. His pillars, or Herms, could once be seen everywhere in Greece, by the roadside and in the villages and cities. Each showed a head and an erect phallus which was adored and anointed with wine and oils by the local people. Occasionally young women would offer their virginity on them, a remnant of the same ritual prevalent in earlier Phoenicia.

Hades, the dark and silent God of the Greek underworld abducted his own niece, the daughter of his sister Demeter, and took her to be his queen. This cycle of events became the basis of the Eleusinian Mysteries. Hades has often been interpreted as a Greek form of Satan ruling over Hell, but this is not true. He simply ruled over those who had died and his kingdom held no punishments.

Probably the most sexual of all Greek Gods was Dionysius, the God of wine and sexual pleasure. His mysteries were celebrated with orgiastic rituals and drunkenness. His Roman counterpart Bacchus was worshipped by women with wild and excessive behaviour. The Bacchantes were dangerous to meet when they were in the power of their rite, as Pentheus found to his cost.

Pan or Priapus was worshipped mainly in country areas and especially at harvest time. He was seen as the protector of flocks and wild animals. At the same time he was noted for his wanton behaviour with human women and nymphs.

# Rome

All forms of worship gradually slide into decline and decay, nothing lasts forever. Rome became the most decadent of all the ancient civilizations – as great as it had been, so as low did it fall. By the end, the early purity of the festivals in honour of the phallus and the vulva had gone for good. The debaucheries of its rulers became a top-heavy weight and Rome fell, dragging with it the then civilized world and opening the doors to the Dark Ages.

Rome had always been a city where prostitution had flourished, fed by the appetites of both men and women. There were many different grades of this ancient profession and the women who practised them were by no means all from the lower levels of society. The highest grade was that of the *Delicatae*, the kept women of the wealthy and prominent men. Next were the *Famosae*, usually the daughters and even the wives of wealthy families who simply enjoyed sex for its own sake. Then there were the *Dorae*, who habitually went naked even in the town and by contrast the *Lupae*, or she-wolves, who plied their trade under the fornices or arches of the old temples, bridges, and the Colosseum. It is from this word that we get 'fornication' as an expression of debased sex. It was one of these lupae, called Laurentia, who found the twins Romulus and Remus and fed them, saving their lives. The *Elicariae* were the bakers' girls who sold the phallus-shaped cakes in the markets and earned a little extra on the side. *Copae* were the serving girls in taverns and inns who could be hired as bedmates for the night by travellers, and the *Noctiliae* were the nightwalkers. Add to these the *Bustuariae*, *Blitidae*, *Forariae* and *Gallinae*, and you will get some idea of how low Rome sank.

# India

The Triple God of India is the Trimurti, consisting of Brahma, Vishnu and Shiva. Each God is one with his consort, forming not three but six deities. This links back to the Hebrew symbol of the six-pointed star as being the universe in total balance. For the Indians sex was the highest form of worship and their Gods used it to maintain the balance between the universe and chaos.

# Sex in the Modern World

Today sex is a paradox. In many ways it is flaunted in full view, in others it is hidden away as if it were something shameful. Our society is divided into several groups: the prudes, the shameless, and those for whom sex is meat and drink. For a very few it is still the sacred fire of life.

## Clothing

Modern clothing varies from month to month; what is in fashion today has disappeared in a few weeks. Always it has followed the way that men see women.

In medieval times women shaved their eyebrows, plucked out their lashes and wore heavy dresses that made them look desirably pregnant. For the men the fashion was decorated codpieces that (usually) lied about their owner's attributes! Sixteenth-century women had panniered skirts and wooden corsets for a narrow waist and a wide hip line, matching the men's padded doublets and tight-fitting hose. The seventeenth century lowered the neckline for women almost, and in some cases, right to the nipples, while the men wore silk and lace and periwigs. By contrast the Puritans covered everything up to the neck!

The 1800s brought high-waisted, neo-classical dresses in fine silks and cottons, worn with little underneath and wetted with lavender water to make them outline the body. Men wore tight pantaloons, knee breeches and make up! By the nineteenth century men made do with suits not too far removed from our own day, but the ladies had changed shape again and were now in crinolines, one of the most awkward shapes ever invented for sitting in. Edwardian times saw the arrival of the full-busted lady with a bustle and hats the size of carriage wheels, then the First World War brought all that to an end and the twenties saw in the 'flapper' with knee-high skirts, flat chests, and a diabolical line in underwear known as directoire knickers. From there it was a short step to mini skirts and the constantly changing fashions of today. Bosoms and hips have disappeared and returned with bewildering rapidity, but underneath there is still *woman*.

## Advertising

To induce people to buy anything today it seems it has to be sold with sex as a carrot – soft drinks, perfume, soap, cars, houses and even insurance. The phallic emblem has returned and the connotation is unmistakable as the young nubile girl tips her head back and drinks from a bottle. Chocolate is sold with the aid of a beautiful woman in her underwear suggestively sliding a bar of the merchandise between her lips. The soap and deodorant and toothpaste ads make sure you get the message that unless you use their product you cannot win a mate. Even coffee and liqueurs are sold by appealing to the romantic in us that longs for the two performers in a British advertisement to get it together. Smell different, taste sweeter, look slimmer, travel further, live faster – we can have it all so long as we buy what the advert people tell us to buy, and sex is the motivation.

## Life-styles

The horse was once the preferred method of abducting your woman, now it is the Porsche, the Ferrari and the Lamborghini, if you are really into wish-fulfilment. If not then any small(er) car will do. Either will be an unconscious extension of your lover's physical attributes. Other items also serve this purpose: a woman's lipstick advertises a second and hidden mouth; her handbag is a symbol of her self, her secret womb where her private and personal treasures are kept. Even if you are a modern feminist with the ability to make your own way in the world, even if you are an independent man not looking for a wife and mother for your children, all these ancient impulses are working inside you. Fight against them and you end up with enough neuroses to choke a cat. Work with them, acknowledge them, but set them aside and they will lie quietly and sleep.

If you do not enjoy sex, well that's too bad, it's good for you, like spinach, but your creative power will not go away. Use it in another manner, but always creatively. You cannot get rid of it with cold showers, but if you turn to a creative outlet, it will get used up safely. How about trying painting, writing, photography, gardening, sewing, embroidery, cookery, bricklaying, burnt poker work, and/or taxidermy?!

We live in a world so different from that of the ancient peoples that their reaction if they were brought up to our time cannot possibly be imagined. Faced with a car, a train, a jet or even something totally simple like a bar of soap or a toothbrush, they just would not be able to cope. The simplicity of their time has been lost forever and with it a kind of innocence. Their idea of sex was, like their lives, simple. It was there, it was immensely enjoyable, you used it, often. What a lot we have lost.

Throughout the recorded history of the world and its religions the power of sex has been a motivating force, even if not recognized as such. It has been lifted high and cast down to the lowest point by humanity, but it has never ceased to be, of itself, the supreme gift of the Creator.

# Part 2
# PROTECTION AND PREPARATION

# 6. SYMBOLS OF CONCENTRATION IN SEXUAL MAGIC

## Sacred Locations

A sacred location is anywhere where magic or ritual (not always the same thing) takes place. Some locations are very old and have been in use for thousands of years. Others are comparatively recent, and yet others are brand new, temples and locations that have been consecrated for magical use by people who know what they are doing.

Examples of the first kind would be Stonehenge, Avebury, Castlerigg Circle, Dinas Emrys and the Rollrights. You would find the second in places such as old disused churches and chapels which in most cases have been de-consecrated and are used for meeting places, recording studios and film sets, or which are part of an estate and have been left unused to become romantic ruins. Alternatively the sacred location might be a place of great beauty that over many years has become ensouled by a Deva, or a grove of trees planted a couple of hundred years ago which has been used by magical groups for a long time.

The last group is your own temple, if you have built one, or the room in which you usually work magic, meditate or study. You do not have to have a custom-built temple in which to work. You can, if all else fails, work any ritual in your head. Ninety per cent of those who will read this book will be using their own home, mostly the bedroom and occasionally the living or dining room. This is sufficient so long as you observe a few rules.

Cleanliness is always the first need. Working magic makes a good excuse to spring clean the room and perhaps paint or paper it, though the latter is not essential. Always make sure your bed is clean – hoover your mattress to get off the dust. *Never* put your shoes or any outdoor clothing on your bed, for they pick up all sorts of things from the outside and I mean all sorts. Lay them on the place where you sleep and anything will cling to it. Your bed has a special importance, especially so when working sexual magic. It is a place where you are vulnerable and relaxed, where your imagination has built up forms and desires over the years. It is where you curl up when you feel ill, tired, desperate, unhappy, angry or sad; it is where you make love. You do not need outside influences coming in to this vulnerable place.

Fresh flowers in a room while you are doing ritual is fine and can add a great deal to the atmosphere, but please take them out before you sleep. Old wives' tales say they take up the oxygen from the room, but what they do as well is attract astral forms and shells. If you put flowers and candles in a room where there is a coffin you are likely to get an apparition, for the energy given out by flowers and light acts like the human energy of a psychic medium. If you sleep with flowers in a room you are more likely to bring astral forms close to you. If you want them close, alright, but if you would rather sleep alone . . . take them out.

If you can, put a dimmer switch on the wall, or else buy some darker shade for your bedside lamps and cover them with different coloured scarves to give subtle shades of light. Do not use an aerosol in a room where you are working magic, for its odours and chemicals will not mix with the oils and incenses you are using and could react with them on the subtle levels. Before a working take down anything that may possibly distract your attention from the ritual. Pictures are an obvious thing here.

The protection of your working space is very important, and it should be attended to before anything else when preparing for the rite. Any clearing and opening rite will suffice, what matters is that it is done. Again, make sure that the closing rite is performed when all has been done. The alternative is the Cord of Power. For this you will need a piece of brand new cord or rope, finger thick, and the exact measurement of your room. Measure carefully all around each side of the room. You do not need to go into oddly-shaped corners, but measure straight across them – this includes window indents and the doorway. Bind the two ends together either with a metal band or by tying them together tightly.

Place the cord around the room, going behind the furniture so that it lies flat against the walls. If you are situated to the four quarters, tie or work into the cord at the eastern point one only of the following: a piece of topaz crystal, a piece of unflawed rock crystal, a piece of consecrated wood like a miniature wand, such as a live wood wand, a small coin painted with gold paint, or a small figure of an angel symbolizing the Winged Man. All these are symbols for the east and the rising sun.

At the south in the same way use a piece of red jasper, a small figure of a lion the size of a charm to symbolize the Winged Lion of the South, or a miniature sword or a heart. In the west use a charm in the form of an eagle, a piece of lapis or turquoise, or a fish. In the north put an onyx, a bull, a corn dolly or a silver coin. This cord must be consecrated in the way you would consecrate any magical implement with earth, water, fire and air. Its intention is to protect in the four directions, plus from above and below. It should be splashed with holy water, censed with incense, sprinkled with salt and breathed upon nine times, then placed in its own bag to be kept clean. If this is placed around the room just before starting any ritual it will set up a ring of protection around the room until it is taken up again.

If you are using an outdoor location clean it of any rubbish, paper and glass, pace out as much ground as you will need and then cleanse it with incense, water and salt mixed together. Those who will be using these rituals will be trained enough to know how to do this, so I will not bother to write it out in full. Always leave an outdoor place clean and tidy. If it is already a sacred site please check to see what kind of work has been done there in the past, as it may clash with what you propose to do. If so, find another place.

I would advise against doing this kind of work in a place where any form of sacrificial work may have been performed, even if it took place thousands of years ago. Sex magic makes you very vulnerable while you are actually joined in union.

# The Five Senses in Sexual Magic

Sensuality is not confined to the genitals – it encompasses all the senses, and especially that of smell. We will take each one in turn.

## Sight

How the loved one looks is coloured by how one thinks of him or her. Beauty, they say, is in the eye of the beholder, and that is true. It means different things to different people and to different races. What we are concerned with here is that you present to your lover and magical partner yourself at your best. This means a clean body, clean hair and nails, and sweet breath. It also means clean clothing (where it is going to be worn). This applies not only to the day of the ritual but should mean every day, and especially during the week prior to the rite. Slopping around in any old thing is not going to make it easy for your partner to make love to you when the time comes.

Make up is not part of the ritual requirements: you will not need false eyelashes, lipstick, nail polish or anything on your face but soap. You need to be your own true self at this time. The sight of a lover clean, fresh, and eager is the best kind of aphrodisiac.

## Sound

Noise can be very distracting in this kind of work. Thick curtains can block out most of the outside noise, and if needed a baffle can be made of thick cork boarding or even thick cardboard. Noise inside can be harder to deal with, so feed the cat/dog and take it out beforehand, make sure your windows do not rattle and above all take the phone off the hook, or put on the answer phone.

Music during a ritual should be just loud enough to be heard, but not enough to distract. Choose your music carefully according to the ritual and its mood. Holst's *Planet Suite* will provide some lovely pieces – Venus, Mercury, perhaps Neptune according to taste – or try Debussy's *Clair de Lune* or *Le Bateau*, Beethoven's *Moonlight Sonata*, or Roderiguez's *Spanish Concerto for Guitar*. Though the title may put you off, listen to Ravel's *Pavane for a Dead Infanta* – its lyrical style may be something you can use. For the first ritual I would always suggest Debussy's *L'Après-Midi d'un Faune*. It reeks of heat, laziness and sensuality. Bob Stewart's psaltery music would be good for the Ritual of the Hawthorn Tower and probably for the Moon Cup. It is a question of taste and mood. *Please* do not choose loud rasping music, it will totally destroy what the ritual is building up.

## Touch

At any time a sensual massage will put either partner in the mood for these rituals. The oils that have been put together by Golden Lotus have been blended specially for these rituals and contain nothing but pure essences. The same goes for the accompanying incenses.[1]

Touch should always be light and caressing at first, then progressing to a firmer and deeper pressure. A light caress is an invitation, a harder pressure is a claiming.

Use the whole of the body to touch your partner. The rub of a man's chest hair against a woman's breasts is highly erotic for both of them. The touch of a woman's leg moving up and down and then entwining with her partner's can raise the blood pressure several points. Even the weight of a man on the woman's body or vice versa can be made into a kind of massage.

[1] Golden Lotus Products have produced a complete range of oils and 11 incenses specially created for the rituals in this book. They are obtainable from Golden Lotus, Amsterdamweg 164, 1182 HK–Amstelveen, Holland or from the UK agent, Dusty Miller, Cudgelmaster, 14 Weston St, Strood, Kent, ME2 3EZ, UK.

Remember there are places where your lover's body is very tender and easily bruised, hurt or even scratched. A woman's breasts and nipples should always be treated gently unless she indicates the need for a firmer pressure. The underside of the breasts, the backs of the knees and the soles of the feet all have vital nerve endings that can be used in erotic massage. The inner thighs and the labia are thin-skinned, so keep your nails trimmed close, and when touching or caressing the clitoris make sure you are in the right place. A surprising number of men do not know where it is. Ask your partner to show you, to place your hands and fingers where she wants them.

A man's body can take a firmer touch, but remember his nipples are just as sensitive: don't bite too hard.

The tongue is an organ capable of touch and taste, and it even helps us to smell. It is a miniature penis and clitoris, capable of arousing your mate to a point where the four-minute warning would go unheard. If you think stroking the back of her knee sends her up the wall, try licking it!

The testicles are vulnerable, so even in fun do not hit, punch or kick them. They do however respond to the hands and tongue and if you have long hair it is worth winding it round the penis and slowly sliding it round and round to watch him go out of his head. Body hair can be pulled (gently), and chest hair is nice to sit on and wriggle! If you haven't tried it, don't knock it.

## Taste

Oral sex, it seems, has only been discovered lately by most Westerners, but in the East and in the Mediterranean cultures it has been used for as long as sex has been around.

Skin not only has different textures, it has different tastes. Before, during and after sex it differs in taste quite markedly. The palms of the hands can be very salty – animals like to lick human hands because of this. The taste of genital fluids can vary with what you have eaten over the past 24 hours. So please not too much garlic the day before a ritual! Some women do not object to the taste or smell of semen, others steadfastly refuse to contemplate oral sex. *Never* force your partner into doing something he or she does not like doing: it is not a loving thing to do. Sometimes a partner will get so wound up that on impulse they will touch or taste in a way they have not wanted to do before. Then let them do it, but do not make a fuss about it afterwards. They may not even have realized what they have done.

Wine and fruit or something sweet by the bed is always a bonus when making love. Chocolate or honey can be smeared on some interesting places and licked off again. A piece of fruit shared between lovers can become unbelievably erotic. Read 'The Song of Solomon' and see how many times the Beloved is compared to food and drink and you will understand the sexual power of taste.

# Smell

Of all the senses the sense of smell is the most important to the sexual act. The olfactory nerves go straight back into the mid-brain or limbic system, the only sense to do so without some kind of transformer. The mid-brain holds all the cards where sex is concerned, for it is here that the hormonal changes are triggered that cause puberty, the menopause and labour contractions, as well as stimulating erections in the male and vaginal secretions in the female. In the lower animals the sense of smell is vital in the seeking out of mates. A male moth will fly an incredible number of miles to a female, following the faint scent trail she had laid down.

We all have our own personal body odour, but with the insistence of today's society that we all smell the same it is very difficult to discern it. Try sniffing a dress or jacket worn by a member of your family and you will find it holds a definite smell, musky but not unpleasant. Once you have smelt this, you should be able to pick out of a heap of clothing the item belonging to that person. Even today, after thousands of years of disregarding our sense of smell, a human being can trace a scent of one part to many thousands.

The use of perfume has been known since the time before Babylon and today it is a world-wide industry. It is pleasant to use scent, and it does have an effect on the male population, but the natural scent of the body should also be allowed to have its time of usage.

Those parts of our body where the personal odour is strongest are usually those parts that are considered 'not nice to touch': the genitals, the cleft of the buttocks and the area around the anus, the vagina, the testicles and penis, the armpits and the soft skin below the ears, the space between the breasts on a female, the small of the back in a male. All these are places where the body scent is strongest and the most erotic. This is why I say do not use scent during the rituals. Unscented soap and water are enough to clean the skin and will allow the body perfume to come through.

Do not be afraid to smell your partner's body. Use the nose like the delicate instrument it is: breathe out all the way, then take in short sniffs until the lungs are full, then breathe out again and repeat. By taking in short bursts of air you will be able to track the scent more clearly.

Dr Septimus Piesse was a famous French perfumer who

invented something he called the 'odophone' or 'science of perfume harmony'. He arranged various scents along the lines of
musical notes, insisting that to form a true bouquet the scents
used should be harmonized with each other. I have taken the
following examples from O.A. Wall's book *Sex and Sex Worship*:

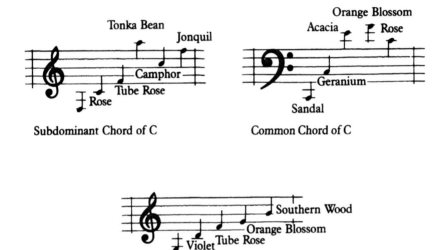

There is room for a whole book on the science of scent and
sexual behaviour, but I have not the space to do it justice here. I
can only say that the effect of scents and perfumes in magical
ritual is a much neglected area.

# Symbols of Concentration in Sexual Magic

Symbols in magic are taught right at the beginning of one's
training; symbols are basics. However when specializing in one
area of magic, as this book does, it is important that the symbols
pertaining to that area are made clear. The following is a list of
male and female symbols that can be used in meditation during
the week before each ritual.

# Male

The Pillar, the Upright Stone or Menhir.
The Tree.
The Mountain.
The Rod or Wand.
The Sword.
The Lingam.
The Lightning Flash.
The Fig Leaf (its trefoil leaf symbolizing the two testes and the penis).
The Staff.
The Lion.
The Unicorn.
The Stallion.
The Hunting Horn.
The Dagger or Athame.
The Caduceus.
The Hammer.
The Sandal.
The Number One.
The Upward-pointing Triangle (this follows the pubic triangle of the male body hair).
The Tau Cross.
The Egyptian Tet and Djed Pillars.
The Cockerel.
The Tower.
The Herm.
The Sun.
The Flute.
The Arrow.
The Sign of Mars.

# Female

The Shell.
The Yoni.
The Grove or Grotto.
The Lily.
The Moon.
The Star.
The Downward-pointing Triangle (the *mons veneris*).
The Cup.
The Dove.
The Cow.
The Oval.
The *Vesica Pisces*.
The Ring.
The Rose.
The Girdle or *Zona*.
The Spindle or Distaff.
The Sistrum.
The Circle.
The Hour-glass.
The Lute.
The Loom.
The Lake/Ocean (or any body of water).
The Sign of Venus.
The Pearl.
The Peacock.
The Basket/Bowl.
The Tomb.
The Cauldron.
The Lotus.
The Scabbard.
The Holed Stone.
A Font.
A Garland.
A Corn Dolly.
A Digging Stick (African).
A Loaf of Bread.
A Cave.
A Boat.

There are of course many more, and everyone should keep a file of pictures of symbols that can be added to as one has need. There are many excellent books available on symbols and symbology.

# 7. THE PREPARATION OF THE PRIEST AND PRIESTESS

The undertaking of a complete series of rituals around a central theme is not one to go into lightly. There needs to be a sense of dedication about it, and a good deal of thought put into it. In the Catholic Church there is a set of prayers known as a 'novena'. This is usually, though not always, said for another person to help them in a crisis or to obtain something they need. A circle of rituals such as these will bring about a similar grace and certainly they will bring a couple much closer together and their bonding will be stronger.

The rituals themselves have been carefully thought out. Some of them may not look at first glance as if they are all that sexual in content – but you will soon learn that a ritual of sexual magic does not have to read like soft porn to be highly effective. I promised myself when I started to write them that I would call a spade a spade and I have done that. What you need to do is to read the whole thing through and ask yourselves, can we do it? Should we do it? Do we need to do it? When you have answered those questions you can start the preparations.

I would suggest that you both start with at least a month of meditations on *why* you wish to undertake what will be almost a full year of rituals. Also meditate on your own sexuality and ask your inner self questions concerning it. Better to get all these things cleared up before rather than during the rituals. For both of you I advise a frank and open discussion on any aspect of sexual activity that may cause problems. For instance, is the man having any difficulties with maintaining an erection, or with premature ejaculation, or even a lack of sexual drive? The rituals are not designed to cure these things – though they may well have some beneficial effects – they are meant to draw the couple closer to their own inner divinity.

The woman should ask herself if she is going to be able to go through the rituals at a fairly steady pace without resorting to the 'headache' excuse. I have found in my own magical work over the years that there are times when, having arranged a ritual, I find myself more and more reluctant as the day goes on to do it. My mind can find a dozen excuses for not doing it and I can get very tetchy about it. However, invariably those are the rituals that go better than any others. I tell you this because it is a syndrome that I often get asked about and it may well manifest during these rituals.

While I think everyone should have the freedom to change little things in a ritual to suit their particular temperament, I think to tamper with these too much will unbalance them. That might cause difficulties in the rituals still to come. The domino effect would come into play and the last one could well give you trouble.

Each of you should prepare yourselves in the way you think fit. After all, I am assuming that you are not novices and have a fair idea of how to prepare for a year of high level work. If you do not, then put the book away until you do. Make the robes you will need well before time and sew them with love. Consecrate them with incense and put them away with scented herbs placed about them. If special things are needed make them in the same way and put them away also. Do everything in a quiet deliberate manner and without rushing. There is no set time for these rites, you can do one a month or one every two or even three months. Remember to record your thoughts, your feelings, and the results, if any, on each ritual.

Where other people are needed for a certain part make sure they are trustworthy and competent. Make sure you are both healthy when you begin the rituals. If you are run down or over-tired and stressed they will make you even more so, for they call on a lot of energy. Time the rituals so they will not clash with the woman's menstrual cycle. While many women feel stronger at that time, others do not as their body is directing energy elsewhere.

If you have children you will need to have someone look after them, overnight if possible, while you are working the rituals. If this is not practical and they are likely to wake up and come looking for you, it would be better to delay the work until they are old enough to sleep through or, if they wake, to understand they must not interrupt you.

The oils and incenses that have been made specially for use with these rites are blended from pure essences. Some of them may contain three or more dozen different scents and materials. Though they are more expensive than some, you will not need as much because of the purity.

Where I have specified a certain number of things like fruit, wine and flowers, etc, use what you have and what you can afford. These are suggestions, nothing more. I have listed all the books I have used for reference in this work. Most of them are unfortunately out of print, but a good library may be able to get them for you. My own collection of books on sexual magic and other areas of the mystical and erotic has taken me many years to accumulate without even knowing why until this book began to take shape in my head.

Please do not attempt these rites if you have quarrelled, or are thinking of parting, or even if you have had a bad day and had a row on the morning of the day you are working one of them. The rites are not for propping up failing marriages or bringing together people who should be apart. If you have the right training you will understand when you read them that each one has many levels and can be worked on any of those levels with very different results. The more you prepare yourselves the better they will work. What you receive from them may be more than you had hoped, and some of you may understand them on even more levels at the end.

# Invocations and Prayers

The offering of prayers and invocations to the God(s) of our choice is a practice as old as humanity. Some of them are beautiful beyond belief and could, like Akenaten's *Hymn to the Sun*, be spoken in any house of worship throughout the world. Those to be found here come from many sources and can be used for almost any type of ritual you may come across. All I would counsel is that you speak them with reverence, no matter if they call upon an aspect of the divine you may not acknowledge. They are all praising that which created the universe and all within it. It, i.e. God, has many names; it is enough that It is.

## Litany
There is no more parting of the ways,
The many have become the One.
I am but a part of one whole, for alone I am nothing.
Together with the One I am all things.
I remain immovable within that place destined for me,
I am part of the great symmetry.
I am responsible for the whole as it is for me.
We are brothers, we are sisters, we are one.
If I am cast down, they shall lift me up,
If one shall go against them I will be their shield.
I shall travel towards the Light and be not afraid,
In the darkness I shall be comforted.
I will rest in the sanctuary of the Light,

I will sleep in the arms of Love.
I am eternal, I am Life.

## Invocation to Yaweh

By His light He hath lighted the morning,
This is He that placed humanity in Paradise.
This is He who made of Nimrod a burning flame
and gifted him with guidance.
All existences are His under His gift.
He possesseth all majesty,
He shines with the power of love.
Behold, all creatures of the earth shall come before Him
and call Him, Lord.

## Prayer for Protection

Now do I call upon the Warriors of Heaven.
Defeat those who would come against me and give me harm.
Turn them back and leave but a sixth part of them.
Come from the north and the south, the east and the west,
and take arms against my foes.
Bring down the mountains upon their heads
and smite the bows from their left hands
and the arrows from their right hands.
Take from them their purpose against me
and deliver me from their wrath.

## Hymn to Ra

Behold thy servants rejoice, and watch thy strength in wonder.
For thou O Ra, hast overcome the wicked.
Thy limbs are pierced with thy sword of light.
Thy fire consumes thine enemies.
Body and Soul are they annihilated.
The Gods rejoice in thy victory.
(Egypt)

## Hymn to Osiris

At the descending of my life's sun I will call to thee.
At the closing of each day I will call to thee.
In all things that need Love, Wisdom and Judgement
I will call upon thee,
For thou art Osiris, the Master of Truth.
(Egypt)

## The Song of the Seven Hathors

They are Seven! They are seven!
In the depths of the ocean they are seven.
In the heights of heaven they are seven.
In the dark spaces between the worlds
and outside of time they were born.

Male and female they are not,
Rule they have, but of prayers they must take heed.
They are seven! They are seven!
Twice over they are seven!
(Egypt)

## Invocation to Ishtar

Adored art thou in every sacred place.
Thou art exalted over all the Gods.
Illustrious is thy name among men,
Lady of ladies and Goddess over all.
The gift of strength is thine for thou art strong.
Heaven and earth lie under thy hand.
Thy ways are just and holy
Look thou upon me with compassion.
Come into this place made for thee,
For behold, it is my heart.
Hear thy servant and harken to my voice
Be merciful, Lady, and appease my sorrow.
(Babylon)

## Invocation to Iacchus

Thou that dwellest in the shadow of great glory stay beside us.
We have come to thee to dance in thy meadow.
O Iacchus, let thy brow toss its fruited myrtle wreath
We are thine, O happy Dancer
Come and guide us
Let the mystic measure beat, come riot with holy feet.
Free and holy all before thee
While the graces three adore thee.
Thy mystae wait the music of thy feet.
(Greece)

## The Magician's Statement of Intent

I am the priest (priestess) of the Gods
I come before thee ....... (name of deity)
In thy greatness I pray thee receive me
Add thy pure voice to mine
Add thy magical power to mine
Add the strength of thy hand to mine.
This is my intent ....... (state intent)
Let it be, let it be, let it be.

## To the Great Mother

Thou of the gentle hands and quiet voice,
hear Thy daughter.
Thou of the endless strength and deep joy,
bend to Thy supplicant.

In all Eternity Thou art there for the weak,
in the Night of Time Thou art a light.
How shall I not come to Thee who art my Mother.

## To Isis

Silver-footed One, come to me with quiet steps
In the temple of my heart.
Lift up thy voice and call my name that I may know Thee
And rejoice in Thy presence.
In my sadness comfort me, in my happiness share with me.
At my birth Thou wast there, at my death wait for me.
Most glorious of women, most tender of mothers,
I am Thy handmaid, bless me.

# 8.  THE POWER OF THE SERPENT

The snake has had a bad press since the Bible came up with the story of the Garden of Eden. The two most common phobias concern snakes and spiders. Yet snakes are relatively harmless if left alone, they menace only if they are frightened and bite only in self-defence.

The serpent has been considered a symbol of sex since the beginning, for knowledge of the good and bad aspects of creative power was the gift of the apple, itself considered to be an aphrodisiac in medieval times. The elongated form of the snake and its ability to rear up gave it a similarity to the erect penis, and both Freud and Jung have written about this symbolism in their books on psychology. Twined about a rod, the snake speaks of sexual passion fully aroused, and we see this in both the Caduceus of Hermes and in the Staff of Aesculapius. Originally the bishop's crozier had a serpent wound around it, something that has been forgotten of late.

Snakes are also a symbol of eternity and immortality, and the serpent holding its tail in its mouth is well known in the occult world. The Jews wandering in the desert after their exodus from Egypt were plagued by venomous snakes, but were 'cured' by the erecting of a tau cross on which a serpent had been crucified. I think that it was probably more than that, for if the snake is a symbol of passion and these desert snakes were termed 'fiery' by those that were bitten, it would appear that what was really troubling the wanderers was an excess of sexual fervour that had probably led to some form of venereal disease. As the snake was also held to have healing properties, this seems a likely reason for the raising of the preventative symbol.

The worship of the serpent was prevalent in many early civilizations. India, Egypt and the North American Indians all saw something holy and divine in the snake and considered it a symbol of knowledge and wisdom. In contrast St Patrick drove all the snakes out of Ireland!

In passing it is interesting to note that some of the early Christian fathers – Justin, Gregory of Nyssa, Augustine and others – held that God had made a mistake when He created man *and* woman. If, they said, Adam had refrained from sexual congress with Eve it would have been a just rebuke to God (how does one rebuke one's Creator?) and would have compelled God (not something I would care to do!) to invent a harmless method of reproduction that did not involve sex. This goes to show how bigoted and repressed such early teachers were against women and sex. Unfortunately they had great influence in their time and it still has a hold.

The power of the serpent Goddess called the *Kundalini* is gradually becoming better known among western occultists, however, and I urge strongly, unless you have been taught Tantra yoga by one who is a Master, leave it alone. There are some western exercises loosely based on the serpent fire which can be used quite safely – you will find some of them in this chapter, and I have provided a ritual based on its God forms – but it is a complex study. To do justice to it one needs to go to an expert. I am not an expert. I have a great respect for it and for what it stands for, but I cannot teach it, I can only adapt some of the less powerful aspects and make them more accessible to western students. The practice of Tantra takes many years of hard work and many books have been written about it in the West. Most of them can be dangerous. Some are little more than an excuse for sex with different partners – something certainly not done according to the rules of Tantra in its native land. The main purpose of Tantra, in the male, is to reverse the power of the seminal fluid and send it up into the brain. In the female it is the menstrual blood that provides the power. The Kundalini, or serpent Goddess, lies in most people coiled quietly around the base of the spine. When she is woken up she begins her ascent to enlightenment. In his book *The Time Falling Bodies take to Light*, W.I. Thompson says:

> . . .whereas the experience of the awakening of the Kundalini in man floods the genitals and causes spontaneous erection in meditation, the equivalent experience in woman causes an ecstatic rapture [that] can be described as an orgasm in the heart, or a giving birth in the heart. The sudden opening of the heart chakra, causes an ecstatic experience of illumination; the heart of the woman becomes the heart of the universe . . . It is for good reason that the sculptor Bernini pictured St Teresa in ecstasy as a woman in orgasm with an angel opening her heart with an arrow.

From this excerpt you can see how powerful an effect the raising of the serpent power can be, and why you have to be cautious when attempting anything along Tantra lines.

The tongue, also considered to be a sexual organ, can be likened to a snake, especially in love play. The interplay between the tongues of lovers can be said to be the mating of the minds, seeing that the tongue is held within the head, whilst the mating of the genitals is that of the body. The snakelike tongue is the equivalent of the snakelike penis, while the soft lips of the mouth echo the equally soft lips of the labia. Looked at in this light, we have been gifted with two sets of genital organs.

# Shakti and Shakta

There are many connotations of these two terms, and in reality they are two types of energy, male and female, but tradition has also made them deities, a supreme male and supreme female who co-operate in a constant sexual interaction. The combination of these two great energies maintains a balance in the universe.

The Trimurti of the Hindu religion consists of Brahma, Vishnu and Shiva. Each is a part of the others, yet each is separate. They may be seen or thought of as Birth, Life and Death. Brahma is the Lord of Creation, Vishnu supports life within that creation, Shiva culminates life and causes it to transcend. Each of the three Gods has a female side, his equal in energy and sanctity. This is his Shakti, his Goddess-partner. She is in no way his inferior or simply another part of himself, she is literally his other half, as he is hers.

Saraswati is the Shakti of Brahma, and with Vishnu goes Laxshmi, while Kali or Parvati is the partner of Shiva. They all have their aspects and their part to play in the balance of life. For a man to say of a woman 'You are my Shakti' is to accept her as an equal in power and influence.

The Shakta is the male of the partnership and corresponds in every way to the female. Therefore a perfect unity is preserved between the two energies.

# Energizing the Centres

Almost everyone is aware of the subtle centres of the body that run from the top of the head to the feet. Each one is a source of a different form of energy that can be tapped and used not only in magical work but in everyday life. Your training will have made you aware of this, but those centres themselves need to be energized, filled up like reservoirs with power from the greater Source. If this is done regularly you should never feel that tiredness that comes from complete exhaustion.

## The Lotus Bud Exercise

Stand with your spine straight, but relaxed and balanced on your feet. Place your hands palms together at the height of your solar plexus. Close your eyes and sink into visual meditation.

From the top of the head there emerges a lotus bud. It opens to reveal its centre, as it does so a shaft of light from the sun strikes down and into the centre of the lotus. The centre of the flower begins to spin. From its centre a thread of light grows downwards reaching for the centre of the third eye. As it does so the centre begins to spin, throwing off sparks of light that fill the whole head and sink into the brain, vitalizing it. Another thread of light emerges and works downwards to the throat centre which also begins to spin, emitting flashes of violet-coloured light that run down both your arms and flow into the fingers.

From the spinning centre the central thread works its way down to the heart centre and sets it spinning like the others. It throws out tiny pulses of blood-red energy that fills the upper part of your body. The thread now grows down to the solar plexus centre and as soon as it touches it, the centre starts to revolve faster and faster. It gives out waves of heat that warm your whole body.

The thread now connects with the genital centre and here the spin is so fast you can see nothing but a blur of deep indigo light that throbs with energy. At last the thread moves down to the feet and earths itself in that centre. It spins more slowly than the others but in turning it gives off a musical sound that is pleasant to the ear. Allow the sun energy to feed the centres for a while until you feel they are fully energized, then slowly withdraw the connecting thread until it leaves the lotus flower. The lotus closes up and withdraws back into the head centre.

## The Dancing Dakinis

A Dakini is a female spirit in Hindu mythology. They are usually depicted as dancing in a highly erotic manner. This exercise is different from the foregoing one and the energy it brings in is more sexual. This makes it a good exercise to do during the days before each ritual. The Dakinis may be pictured as small but perfectly formed women of great beauty, and their dances, although suggestive, are graceful and delicate in their steps and use of the body.

It is best to lie down for this exercise – but not after a meal as you will drift off to sleep. Support the neck, the small of the back, the knees and ankles with rolled towels. Begin with the feet and build in the mind a glowing sphere of reds, browns and dark greens encompassing them. Slowly the colours clear and you see a tiny female form curled up as if asleep within the sphere. She wakes and rises to her feet, holds out her arms, smiles, and begins to dance. Her garments are the colours of the earth and in her dance is all the energy of the changing seasons. She goes through each one. For a man she is the earth itself in woman's form, to the woman she is what the woman herself desires to be. Her dance ends and she sinks down and returns to sleep.

Build the next sphere in the genital area, make it glow with deep violet light swirling round and round. The light clears to show the Dakini sitting cross-legged in the centre. She open her eyes and smiles, then, rising to her feet, she begins to dance. She dances the story of man and woman and the universe of love, and as she twists and turns she drops her veils one by one until she is naked, offering herself to your eyes. To the man she is desire, to a woman she is love. She sinks down into contemplation and closes her eyes.

Build the next sphere in the solar plexus. Visualize a fiery sun full of heat and flame. Its colours are red, orange and yellow, and its Dakini is dressed in golden armour and carries a sword and a shield. She is a warrior maid and her dance is full of energy and spirit. She raises the body heat and keeps our courage high when we feel afraid. To a man she is strength, to a woman she is power. Her dance ended, she stands tall and straight and salutes you with her sword.

The next sphere is the heart centre, coloured in rose and amber gold. Its Dakini is dressed in those colours and her dance is soft and gentle and full of tenderness. She arouses in humanity the love of others, the love of the smaller weaker ones and those placed in our care. To a man she brings gentleness without weakness, to a woman she gives a true heart. She closes her dance with a gesture of enfolding a form in her arms, then sinks down into sleep.

The next sphere, the throat sphere, is lavender in colour and swirls in quick circles. The Dakini is light on her feet and darts to and fro, leaping and twisting. Her gestures are quick and nimble and she moves so swiftly it is hard to watch her. Her eyes are full of laughter and she is dressed in silver from head to foot. Her gift to both man and woman is the gift of speech and the silver tongue. Finally she stops, motionless but poised ready to begin again.

Next a sphere of emerald green beckons to us from the Third Eye position. In its depths we see a slender figure moving slowly as if in a trance. Her hands and arms create visions and dreams each more beautiful than the last. She is the giver of hope and visions, of glimpses into the future and the past. She offers clear sight and insight as her gifts. She never sleeps but waits until needed.

Finally we reach the last sphere, that of the fontanelle. It is the colour of pale gold and in its depths we see a Dakini lying as if asleep. She is the most beautiful of all and her gift is that of wisdom, but before she can bestow it, she must be awakened. To do that we must find the hidden path into the sphere and there are few who will succeed.

# Part 3

# THE RITUALS OF THE TREE OF ECSTASY

# INTRODUCTION

The last part of this book is purely practical and comprises the rituals themselves. Each one corresponds to the *Keynote* of a particular sphere on the Tree of Life, hence the title of the book itself. This is simply to give an overall pattern to the rituals and make it easier to grasp the idea of the many different types of power that fuel them. Thus the Rite of Pan will correspond to the sphere of Malkuth, while the Calling of a Soul will align with the sphere of Binah and so on.

You will find that these rituals are exactly what I promised they would be, i.e. magical rites of sexual polarity. Such rituals are also a very potent form of High Magic and not to be worked lightly. Neither are they to be demeaned by using them simply for the self-gratification of sexual intercourse and giving nothing to the Gods. To do so will be to invite upon yourselves a swift and exacting retribution, for you do not use the creative force of the cosmos under ritual conditions for your own human lust. The dedication and concentration of purpose is what sets these rituals apart from anything you may have been told or have read about in the past.

Each and every ritual that follows is an *act of worship* that uses a primal and mighty power, a power that is locked up in every human being. When understood and used in a balanced, harmonious and reverent way, this power can lift men and women to the very portals of divinity; when abused it can become the cause of a personal *fall from grace*.

Besides establishing the Keynotes of each ritual the pattern of the Tree of Life has been used for a second purpose, and that is to symbolize a spiralling ascent towards the perfect union of male and female. These rituals move through the levels from the physical to the emotional, on to the intellectual and finally up to the fully spiritual. Therefore each one represents a step upward, not only in the understanding and usage of the creative power but in the gradually awakening harmony between a man and a

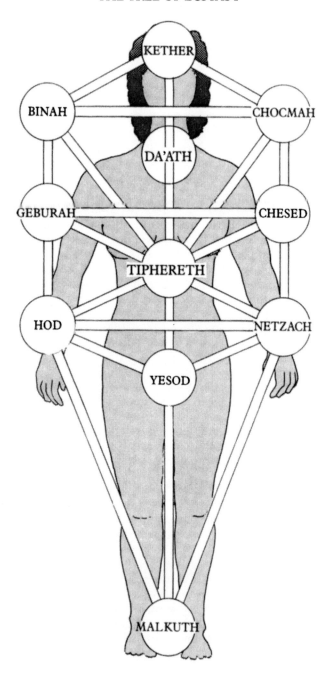

*Figure 2:* The Tree of Life

woman. It is important to realize this from the beginning, or the shifting emphasis of the rituals – some female orientated and some male, with others balanced between the two – can be misunderstood.

Each ritual is complete within itself, and they do not all follow the same tradition. Nevertheless they are linked in other ways to form a coherent path of instruction when followed correctly. The Keynote of its sphere of placement on the Tree together with the inner and higher meaning embodied by the rite itself will act in a similar way to the paths on the Tree of Life. To strengthen that link I have provided short pathworkings to go with each ritual. These may be seen as a means of keeping contact with the higher levels of the pattern yet to be used.

It is essential that the correct pacing of these rituals must be adhered to in the first instance. One per month is the absolute maximum, one every six to eight weeks would be a better ratio. This applies no matter how much experience you have or how long you have been working magic.

If you are doing other magical work as well you must be doubly careful to space the rituals apart. Once you have gone right through them in sequence, you may use them in whatever order you like, applying them to seasons or to specific occasions. Just take care that you match the ritual to the occasion and not the other way around. In other words, do not use the ritual corresponding to Tiphereth for a season or an occasion that would be better served by that written for Netzach.

Each ritual is preceded by a run-up programme. This attunes the body, mind and spirit to the required Keynote. There are specific exercises for this along with a brief outline of the inner meaning and possible outcome of the ritual itself and the God form it employs. The accompanying pathworking can be used as a means of lowering the spiritual, mental and sexual tension during the days after the ritual.

Never lose sight of the fact that humanity was given its sexuality as a divine gift. It is a gift that offers both an open and a hidden path to divinity, for there is so much more to it than personal pleasure and/or the conception of a child, both of which should be seen as gifts within the absolute gift. The act of love is the greatest and most unknowable of all the mysteries for it encompasses birth, life and death within itself. It is also an act of sacrifice, for at the moment of sexual climax each gives themselves up to the other and in doing so receives far more than they give.

Wrapped within the auric vortex of the act each man becomes 'the Primal Sword'. He is at that moment the sacrificial priest that pierces, wounds, fills and pleasures his priestess, making of her something unutterably holy. He offers the living sacrifice of his seed on and within the altar of her body, her womb being the sacred chakra of the feminine principle and therefore every bit as holy and as consecrated as a church, temple, chapel, sacred circle or any place set aside for worship.

We enter a church or any holy place to seek a renewal, a communion or meeting with the unknowable source of all life, we speak of the Church as being *female*, calling it 'Mother Church' 'The Bride of Christ' and so forth. We emerge from such a place with renewed faith, hope and zest for life, having touched the source of life itself. So it is with the act of love: a woman is made holy by the fact that she is a vessel of creation (whether she chooses to be a mother or to use her creative power in another way) and her womb is a chalice into which the wine of life may be poured. Because of this fact rape is not only a crime on the physical level, it is a *spiritual* sin and its aftermath requires a spiritual cleansing and a reconsecration of the sacred chakra if the woman is to feel cleansed and whole within herself again.[1] Just as every man is a priest of love, so every woman becomes 'the Royal High Priestess', the chalice that uplifts, accepts and enroyals her priest, transmuting the seed of life either into a new human being or into an offering of love to the Creator. Either outcome should be considered holy, divine and ineffable.

[1] See The Healing Ritual in the revised edition of my *First Steps in Ritual*, The Aquarian Press, Wellingborough, 1990.

# Ritual 1

# THE RITE OF PAN

## The Programme

Pan is the goat-foot God of foothills, forests and woodland plains, and Old Pan is a pre-chaos being. In the first instance he is seen as the protector and guardian of animal life. He is one of many archetypes termed 'the Horned Gods', an appellation that surprisingly includes the prophet Moses, but unlike Cernunnos and Herne the Hunter, the deer-antlered Gods of the Celts, Pan wears the ram's horns, symbols long associated with the power of fertility and sexuality.

He is therianthropic, half-man half-animal, having the upper torso of a powerful, well-muscled man in the prime of life and the lower limbs and hooves of a goat. He is generally pictured as being bearded with a thick mane of hair brushed back from the forehead, slightly slanted golden eyes, a hooked nose and curving sensual mouth. He is permanently erect and because of this is often wrongly confused with the God form Priapus. For pathworkings and meditational purposes it is best to picture him in his most benign form. I would advise reading a chapter entitled 'The Piper at the Gates of Dawn' from the children's classic book *The Wind in the Willows* by Kenneth Grahame. The description of Pan given there is one of the best you will find anywhere.

Because of his legendary exploits with the nymphs and dryads of his domain as well as his link with the earth and animal kingdom, the goat-foot God is ideal for use in the sphere of Malkuth. He symbolizes the power of sex to both fertilize and pleasure the female in its most primal form. This is the 'garment' taken on by the male principle in the following ritual, while the wild, free aspect of the nature spirits of woods, trees and water can be taken on by the female principle.

The one thing you must remember about this particular God form is that it can change drastically if allowed to get out of hand.

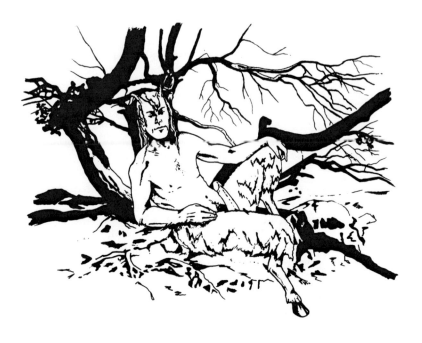

*Figure 3:* Pan *(Paul Hardy)*

Then it becomes the bringer of Pan-ic fear and lust that can cause untold havoc within the psyche. It is because of the need for self-control and inner balance that the rituals in this book (and indeed the book itself) are *not* for the beginner, the unbalanced or the sensation seekers – and there are far too many of the latter in the occult world! Everyone carries their idea of Pan within their deepest self. If the inner Pan is balanced and one's attitude towards the God form is pure and trusting, then it is safe from the terrible fear and rage of which it is capable. If, however, the inner nature is corrupt and unbalanced then the inner Pan becomes he who rips and rends, the bringer of fear.

The older version of Pan is a proto-neolithic archetype and its image may be seen in many of the ancient cave paintings, the most famous of which is 'The Dancing Sorcerer' in Les Trois Frères cave at Lascaux in France. But this pre-chaotic form is also a creative archetype. From it comes the impetus that creates order from chaos and existence out of nothingness. To do this requires a massive burst of creative energy such as that described in the Big Bang theory. The act of sexual union follows the same format even when enjoyed purely for one's own pleasure, but when used in ritual conditions, with both partners fully aware of the forces they are using, then the resulting explosion of directed energy and its power can well be imagined. On a lighter note, the euphemistic use of the word 'bang' to describe a sexual encounter makes one wonder if the sub-conscious mind has its own separate sense of humour!

Begin preparations for the ritual a week ahead by setting aside 15 minutes in the morning and another 15 minutes in the evening. If you cannot do this due to lack of time or self-discipline then postpone the ritual, or any of the rituals, until you can. You cannot play around with sexual magic. In fact, you cannot play around with *any* form of magic, but here you are working with highly volatile creative power, a transmuting energy similar to a nuclear device. Making the earth move is really a very good description of sexually orientated magic!

The daily procedure is as follows: on waking dispense with your pillows and lie flat with arms at sides. Now stretch the legs and feet downwards, feeling the pull right to the tips of the toes. Then do the same with the arms and hands, paying attention to the fingers. Then tip the head back and arch the spine, lifting it off the bed as far as you can so that there is a space between the head and the hips. If you cannot manage so much, then do what you can. The object is to get all the muscles fully stretched and 'alive'. Now relax for a few seconds then repeat again. At this point the exercises for man and woman differ. The female exercises are as follows.

Replace your pillow, place the open palm of the right hand about three fingers depth below the navel, just over the sacred chakra of the womb. Let the other hand lie flat on the left thigh. Now breathe in through the nose and imagine the air as carrying 'light'. Pool it in the heart centre between the breasts. Breathe out through the mouth, pursing the lips in a blowing action, and imagine the inhaled 'light' being forced down the right arm through the palm of the hand and spiralling into the womb in a clockwise direction. In a few moments the chakra will grow warm and may begin to pulse. Do this seven times, then change hands, placing the left palm on the womb and resting the right hand on the right thigh. As you breathe in imagine the energy now spiralling in the centre is flowing into the palm of your hand up

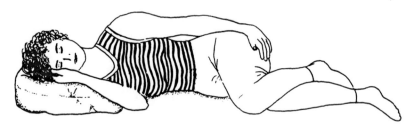

*Figure 4:* Female exercise

the arm to pool between the breasts. On the out breath push the air through the mouth and the used energy is pushed out. Repeat seven times. This simple exercise uses the life energy of *air* (in the East it is called *prana*) to awaken and vitalize the female sacred chakra and to drain away the used energy again.

Lie on your right side with the left knee drawn up, your right hand under your cheek and your left hand on the left thigh (see Fig 4). Breathe in normally and hold for a count of four. With each count tighten the vaginal muscles *without tensing the rest of the body* then breathe out and relax the muscles. Repeat this exercise twice more. This concludes the female morning exercises.

Now for the male exercises. Stretch in the same way as described above, and when this has been done proceed as follows. A man often awakes in the morning with a full erection – this is quite normal as every man well knows, but what you may not know is that the sexual power locked into this erection is the most powerful of all. The body is refreshed with sleep at this time, and particularly the testes, and all the creative power is pooled into the genital area. Breathe in and hold for a count of four. While holding the breath tighten and relax the buttocks once for each count and at the same time use your muscles to lift the scrotum. Repeat twice more. This will strengthen the muscles and tone the scrotum area which can grow slack with age or lack of exercise.

Get up and sit on the edge of a chair, or the bed if it is firm enough. Keep the back straight and allow the testicles to hang freely. Breathe in with short, gentle inhalations, stopping after each little intake. With the first breath mentally send the *prana*-bearing air down as far as the solar plexus, with the second send it down to the lower belly. The third needs to thrust it down to the right testicle, and four sends it across to the left. Now begin to breathe out in the same way, but tighten and lift the scrotum as you do so. The first exhalation sends the used air to the belly, the second to the solar plexus, the third to the back of the throat, and

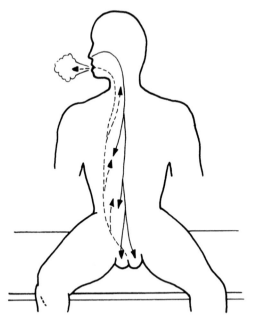

*Figure 5:* Male exercise

the last blows it out through the mouth in a small explosion (see Fig 5).

Repeat this three times, wait a minute or so and then repeat another three times. This exercise cleanses the body right through and empties it of stale energy. Gently massage the scrotum as it hangs down to encourage the flow of new energy. If the erection is still present allow the power to descend of its own accord. The retention of the 'morning power' will add energy to your day. Both the vagina and the scrotum should be bathed in cold or cool water at least once a day, summer or winter, as this stimulates the flow of blood to those areas.

The evening exercise 'the Calling Forth' is a beautiful and gentle way for two people to acknowledge the divinity in each other. After bathing stand naked facing each other, taking the time to really look at each other, to take note of the day's influence on your faces. Does his face seem more tired than usual, or is there the sparkle that comes from facing and overcoming a challenge? Does she wear a gentle smile or can you see signs of an upset in her day? Seek out the little signs and note them, then let your findings dictate your expression of feeling towards your partner.

Link hands and lean forward to greet each other as friends. Let the kiss be light and undemanding, draw back, look again. Lean forward and greet each other as understanding partners who share their lives. Draw back and look a third time and now greet each other as lovers and allow the passion to rise, but keep it under control. Keep holding hands but do not caress each other.

Now the man touches the woman on the head and says to her, 'You are woman.' Pause a moment and think about that, try to understand its full meaning. Touch her forehead and say 'You are understanding.' Again think about its meaning. Now touch the throat: 'You are my link with the spirit.' Pause and think. Touch between her breasts: 'You are my nourishment.' Pause. Touch just below the navel: 'You are the chalice of life.' Touch the opening of the vagina: 'You are the maker of forms.'

Now it is the turn of the woman. She touches the man's head and says, 'You are man.' Pause and think about the statement. Touch the forehead: 'You are wisdom.' Touch his breast: 'You are my strength and my protection.' Pause. Touch his belly: 'You are my warmth.' Pause. Touch the penis: 'You are the fount of life.'

This interchange allows the two partners to acknowledge each other on many levels: as human beings, as the holders of different kinds of strength, as people with different needs and the ability to provide each other with the assuagement of those needs, as spiritual keepers of the life forces, and last but never least, as lovers.

When this interchange is done, take just 10 minutes to meditate on one of the symbols for this ritual, and on alternate days use the pathworking given below. The symbols are as follows: a pine cone, pan-pipes, a ram's horn, a pair of cymbals and a shepherd's crook. The pine cone is a fertility symbol appropriate for Pan, and the pipes are his signature with their lilting, luring music that draws both humans and the birds and beasts to his side. Pan always wears the ram's horns and *never* the deer antlers. The cymbals, while rightly being the instrument of the Bacchantes, can also be seen as symbolic of the wilder sexual side of the woman or nymph, and the crook shows the caring gentle aspect of Pan as the guardian of the forest wildlife.

The last two nights before the ritual itself you can change to the following procedure. Again the exercise is performed nude, but this time just before sleeping. On the first night the woman sits cross-legged on the edge of the bed. If the position is uncomfortable, use the God form position with a cushion beneath the feet to lift them. The hands are cupped over the pubic area with a fresh flower lying in the cup of the hands. The man sits in the same position on the floor in front of the woman, looking up. He contemplates the woman as maiden, wife, and wise woman, as a partner, friend, companion, priestess and lover. After 10 minutes rise up and receive the flower from her hands and a kiss from her lips. Place the flower between you when you sleep. While her partner meditates the woman should mentally go through the stages with him.

On the night before the actual ritual, reverse the positions, the man sitting on the bed, his hands holding either a wand or an athame. The woman sits looking up and contemplating her partner as the youth, the warrior/or the seeker, and the wise man/mage. During this time read all you can about the goat-foot God and his companion nymphs and build up your inner images.

Music can be used with great effect during this ritual. Debussy's *L'Après-Midi d'un Faune* is one of the most evocative, also his suite *La Mer*, and a short piece called *Le Bateau*. 'Venus' from Holst's *Planet Suite* and Georgi Zamfir's pan-pipe music is also excellent. Anything suggesting long hot lazy hours in the sun, or something equally hot and wild in the sexual sense will do. I should not have to remind you that while their music may 'turn you on', artists like The Grateful Dead, The Rolling Stones, and Tina Turner are not ritual material!

The last instruction will not be popular but it applies to all the rituals in this book and is essential to their success. On no account must sexual intercourse take place during the week prior to the ritual. You may look, touch and caress but neither partner must achieve a climax (this applies to masturbation as well), and if this rule is disobeyed you must return to the beginning and go through the procedure again. Why? Because the energy and the inner sexual tension must be allowed to build gradually until it is only just below the surface and under tight control. If you cannot obey this rule, this book and its contents are not for you.

For obvious reasons it is best to plan the ritual for a weekend, provided you can make it quite clear to relatives, family and casual callers that you are completely unavailable. Adjust the answer phone if you have one so that the recording answers after the first ring, and if you have no answer phone, take the phone off the hook, unplug it, or bury it under a pile of cushions. In dire need hang it out of the window!

For the ritual itself you will need the following: ten candles, five dark green and five gold; incense; body oils; a bowl of herbs and crushed leaves mixed with salt; two pottery cups or goblets and some red wine (not white, it must be red and full flavoured, if you are a non-drinker use red grape juice); a basket or wooden bowl filled with fruit – apples, figs, dates, pomegranates, small sweet tomatoes, olives, grapes, peaches/nectarines if in season, strawberries, raspberries, etc. You can add some nuts to the fruit bowl if you like them. If you can, make some homemade bread rolls with coarse wholemeal flour and have a small bowl of honey in which to dip them.

If you cannot afford all of these things then just use two or three, working according to your normal budget. Your incense might be a good quality Dittany of Crete, but you can use crushed bay leaves, rosemary and thyme mixed in with it. The candles can be used about the room in ones and twos, or grouped all together at one point.

Unless you have a temple that can be used, use your bedroom, but make sure you clean it thoroughly. Move out all you can, including the television if you have one in the bedroom, and clear small ornaments, pictures and any extraneous objects away. The room should be pleasantly warm and decorated with leafy branches to give the impression of a woodland setting. If gathered fresh and of mixed variety, they will fill the room with the special scent of trees and sap and crushed leaves.

Strip the bed and cover it with a clean white bottom sheet only, but have a light blanket close to hand, also a Thermos flask of warm water and some small towels. Place a small table either side of the bed and place the fruit, wine, bread and honey on one, and a bowl, the water and towels and the body oils on the other. If you prefer, they may all be placed on one low table elsewhere in the room with cushions scattered around the room. On the bed scatter some flower petals and leaves but make sure they are soft and not uncomfortable to lie on.

As you prepare the room keep the ritual and its intention in mind. You are doing all this with a real purpose – not sex, but a ritual of High Magic. You are preparing to welcome the Great God Pan and his priestess into your home and your hearts. You will assume those God forms and become one with them, offering the ritual and all that it entails as an act of worship to the creative force that permeates the cosmos.

Complete your arrangements in the morning and in the afternoon prepare the room itself. If you have children, arrange for them to stay with friends or relatives. If you want to do the ritual badly enough you will find a way to be alone, and you *must* be alone. Once everything else is prepared, it is time to prepare yourselves.

Fill the bath with warm – but not hot – water, and sprinkle a small handful of sea salt in it and some crushed herbs, but nothing else. Bathe separately, and as you do, think of the words you have said to each other every evening and try to understand the inner and higher meaning behind them as you anoint your bodies with the chosen oils. Finally you come together and, naked except for coronets of flowers, you enter the prepared room. Slowly and reverently light each candle, pausing between each one. Start the music and begin to build the Temple of Pan for your rite.

# The Rite of Pan


## Place on the Tree = Malkuth. Keynote = The Physical Realm.

*The man takes the bowl of leaves, herbs and salt and, taking a small handful, throws it to the east.*

**Man:** I summon the winds of the east to fill this place with the scent of spices from the lands beyond the dawn. Cleanse and make fragrant this place, that our joining may likewise be clean and pure and pleasing to the Great God Pan.

*He turns to the south and throws a second handful.*

I summon the winds of the south to fill this place with the scent of flowers, of rose and jasmine, lotus and moon-flower and warm it with the southern sun, that our joining may be like the fire of the sun itself.

*He turns to the west and throws a third handful.*

I summon the winds of the west to wash this place with the soft rain of heaven, to wash away all thought of self and allow us to join like those drops of rain, without restraint, formless and fluid.

*He turns to the north and throws the last of the herbs and salt.*

I summon the winds of the north to protect and hallow this place with their breath of ice. Behind such white walls we will join in joy and offer that joy to the oneness that will persist throughout eternity.

*The woman goes to the southeast with a small glass of wine and offers a few drops as an offering.*

**Woman:** I am the sacred vase of life, I am the container of joy. I offer that with which I shall be filled to the source of all things through the God form of Pan and Syrinxe his priestess.

*She goes to the southwest, and offers a few drops of wine.*

I am that which endures the flame of birth and causes the gates of life to open to my call. I offer my gift of love to the creatrix of all things.

*She goes to the northwest and offers the wine as before.*

I am the power behind the sun, that power is mine to reflect upon the earth and upon my beloved. To the intention of this rite I offer that power.

*She goes to the northeast and offers the wine for the last time.*

I am life in all its forms. Nothing lives but it comes from me, from womankind. I give and I take and shall do so throughout eternity, but always with love.

*The man and woman sit facing each other in the centre of the room. Slowly they open each psychic centre in turn. First the top of the head glows golden, then the light is drawn down to the third eye centre where it lights up like a tiny sun, then down to the throat where another small sun is lit with an amethyst glow, then to the heart centre where the little sun is blood red, and on to the solar plexus which is the seat of the personal sun and glows gold and amber.*

*Now it differs between man and woman. In the woman the light travels on to the sacred centre of the womb to become a rose-coloured flame, then on to the genitals, taking the form of a star. Finally it reaches the soles of the feet and becomes a green seedling that coils about each ankle. The man draws the light from the solar plexus down to the point between and slightly behind the testicles where it becomes a white flame, then on to the feet which it covers with the semblance of hooves.*

*Now each must build within their heart centres a miniature image of the God form they are invoking: the Great God Pan for the man and the nymph Syrinxe for the woman. When the image is clear – and it must be your idea of the forms – let it grow, filled with the power and the energy of the solar centre until the form fills the physical body. As it fills you, the power and the nature of the immortals will also fill you. Pan is strong and eager, full of life and strength and the need to chase, catch and overcome. Syrinxe is shy, warm, soft and sweet, yet teasing and wanton beneath the shyness. Both are fully aware of themselves and of their hosts.*

*Fill the cups with wine and drink. Look at each other with the eyes of God and nymph. Now Pan dips his finger into the honey and with it draws flower patterns around each of the nymph's nipples, tipping them with honeyed centres. Her mouth is likewise etched with honey; her navel, inner thighs and labia, toes and the tender soles of her feet are all lightly ribboned with the bees' sweet store. The nymph responds in kind, drawing patterns and trails of honey on Pan's body, seeking out the unexpected places – behind the knees, on the hip bone, following the muscle curve to the phallus that awaits its honeyed crown.*

*Pan's intention is to reclaim what he has given and he desires the sweetness on his tongue, but Syrinxe must first be won. Nothing must be hurried at this point, and control must be kept. It is in the flight and the chase that the power of the ritual is built up. Pan is the cosmic lightning flash that seeks to lose itself in the warmth and moistness of the earth, the nymph Syrinxe. Gradually the higher level of Pan and nymph must be brought through. The laughter and the teasing act as a key to open the lower levels, but now the upper levels must be opened. Here the ritual intent become critical, for you must hold and control the desire level, yet keep it open and ready.*

*Syrinxe now becomes the earth itself welcoming the cosmic fire. Pan kneels before her, looking at her not as woman, or even as Syrinxe, but as the open cosmic chalice that his fire must fill. She must call that fire from him, as is her right. The herb-strewn bed is the symbol of the underlying universal matter and it is here that fire and chalice will meet and fulfil their purpose.*

*The nymph kneels on the meeting place of heaven and earth, her arms outstretched to the side, the fragrance of the crushed herbs and leaves and her own body scent acting as added incense for the rite. Pan kneels behind her, his arms alongside hers, their hands linking together. It is almost time.*

*The human bodies and emotional selves must be lost in the greater aspect of that which is now in control. You must make a conscious effort to offer the ecstasy of the union to the Source of Creation, the Greater Pan that was before all things were.*

*Syrinxe bends slowly forward and the body of Pan follows her lead. His arms curve hers inward so she is enclosed and enfolded within the greater male strength, yet knowing her own inner strength is its equal.*

*Because this is a primal blending it follows a primal mating pattern and the phallus enters the vagina from behind. The Gods remain enfolded for a long moment, again testing human control, then the mating begins. In the mind let a great storm begin, feel its rain on your bodies, hear the noise of the thunder, see the flash of the lightning. Ride the storm as one person far beyond the pale meaning of male and female. Together you are the primal parents of earth. Catch the moment just before the final lightning bolt strikes through the melded hearts and bodies and offer everything that is happening to you, everything you are at that moment, to the creative force of the cosmos for its use.* Keep nothing for yourself.

*The moment will hang suspended like an eagle on the wind, then you must allow the God forms to return slowly each to their small image in the heart centre. Slowly again, return to the posture of outstretched arms, linked hands, one kneeling behind the other. Close the centres one by one, starting with the feet. Pull up the thread of light from which they were made until it reaches the genitals, there let it gather up the remnants of the spent force, then flow up again. Stop to collect the force left in the sacred centre of the womb, then continue on and up, collecting whatever force is left from each centre until you reach the head, where the light widens out like a fan. Now it blends with the aura, strengthening it and filling it with the residue of power. Now you may rest.*

*As you do so, allow your minds and bodies to become aware of your surroundings: the scent of the herbs and incense mixing with the normal body scent, the soft light from the candles, the aroma of the branches and leaves, the taste of wine and honey on your tongue and the salt of your sweat, the coolness as your body temperature returns to normal and the sound of the blood singing through your veins. You may just catch an echo of a voice crying, 'Pan, Io Pan, Io Pan.'*

*When you feel ready, eat from the fruit and the bread and honey, and drink the wine. It will help you to close down firmly. You are vulnerable at this time, but the circle will protect you. Sleep if you wish, and in the early morning you will wish to make love in the ordinary human way, delighting in each other and sharing your delight. It is yours, unlike the great sweep of power that you conjured up from within the heights and depths of your psyches earlier. Later still there will be time to wonder. The Rite of Pan has ended.*

# The Pathworking

Under a brilliantly blue sky the sun beats down on a small river winding its way to the sea. On one side of the river there are open grasslands, on the other densely-packed woods. In the middle of the river is a large flat stone, and on it, lying in the sun and half asleep in the fierce heat, lies Syrinxe, a nymph. She has discarded her one thin garment and after bathing in the river has stretched out to let the sun dry her long honey-brown hair.

At first the birds call to each other across the river and among the trees, but as the heat of the day increases they too fall silent and leave the bees to provide the only sound. From time to time a solitary breath of wind brings the scent of sweet grasses and wild herbs growing on the open fields. All is silent and still. The heat presses down and even the river seems to flow more slowly as if finding it too hot to move.

For a long time there is nothing but the sun, the river, the heat and the beautiful Syrinxe immobile on her rock in the sun. When the sound is first heard it is so faint that it seems merely an echo of something long ago. A mere breath of sound, yet the heart pauses in its beat to listen. There is a pause, then it is heard again, just as soft but now it seems to have more substance to it, one can be certain of having heard it hanging on the still air. A third time it comes and this time nearer and more continuous. It comes from the forest and it is the sound of the pipes. The silver cadences flow and dance adding their magic to that of the stillness, again and again they call, dipping and lilting, sometimes sounding like a bird call, and at others a plaintive lullaby that urges the world to sleep and dream under the noon sun. Syrinxe stirs and rolls over on to her belly, sleepily opening her eyes and focusing on her reflection, then her head drops on to her arms and she sleeps again.

A bird wakes up and answers the call of the pipes. They reply, and soon bird and pipes are engaged in a duet of liquid harmony that echoes far and wide. The pipes are much nearer now and the lower notes more discernible to the ear. Syrinxe has woken and sits up to listen. She smiles, knowing full well who is coming. She laughs and hugs her knees, holding her head to one side listening as the pipes concede defeat to the little feathered singer.

There is a pause and now the pipes begin again, so skilfully played that they seem to call a woman's name. 'Syrinxe, Syrinxe,' they say and the nymph laughs again and sits quietly waiting. The piper is now almost in sight and the music loud and clear, but abruptly it stops and silence falls. After a while the nymph lifts her head, frowning at the silence. When it continues she rises to her feet and, shading her eyes, scans the forest for the unseen musician. After a while she jumps down from the rock, forgetting her dress in her curiosity, wades across the river and runs lightly towards the trees. There she stops and peers into the depths of the greenwood as if looking for the elusive piper, but he is nowhere to be seen.

Disconsolately she walks back to the river, but before she has gone three paces a figure leaps from the trees and races after her. Looking over her shoulder she screams, half in fear and half in excitement, and runs like a hare for the river. Pan, for it is he, almost catches her but she is too quick and is now atop her stone in the river, once more laughing and defying him. She knows full well he dislikes running water and will enter it only if there is no other way to get across.

Pan sits down on the bank and begins to play. The pipes urge the nymph to dance, and she does, using the flat rock as her dancing floor. As he plays Pan's bright amber-coloured eyes watch her and his horns catch the sunlight as his head moves to his own music. The muscles on his arms flex and ripple as he moves and his shaggy limbs are splayed at ease on the grassy verge.

Syrinxe too is overcome and begins to wade across the river when a pollen-heavy bee, too laden to fly straight, attempts a landing on Pan's nose. He pauses to lift it gently away and lay it on a flower and in the pause Syrinxe escapes from the music spell and takes to her feet, running downriver through the shallows. Pan runs after her, knowing that he can easily outdistance her. Now the music changes and becomes pleading, it invites and coaxes the nymph to come and play the ancient game of love. Subtly it calls, and the birds and beasts around venture from the forest to hear. Soon they are obeying its command to love and be as one, male with female as was ordained. Syrinxe hears Pan running after her and tries to makes for the deeper water, but he is upon her and lifts her high into his arms, laughing in triumph. She is quiet in his arms, content to be carried towards the trees.

Within the green dome of the forest the heat is less intense and beneath the spreading branches of an ancient tree Pan lays down his precious burden. She smiles and holds out her arms, knowing full well who is the conquered and who the conqueror, for what man has ever outwitted a woman? He lies beside her caressing her rosy skin and kissing each pearl-tipped finger. Two interested rabbits watch curiously until with a wide grin Pan waves them away and they scamper off into the tree roots.

The silence falls once again, the pipes are still, the only music to be heard is the soft sound of Syrinxe sighing as Pan fits their bodies together in the ancient pattern of creation. The heat and silence now take over and the scene fades.

# Ritual 2

# THE RITUAL OF THE MOON CUP

## The Programme

The second ritual might well be termed neo-pagan, but its origins lie in the mysteries of the Old Religion. The basic idea is not new – in its earliest form it probably dates back to around the early 1600s. Here it has been given a modern approach, but the effect is still highly potent.

Yesod is the next sphere after Malkuth. It is concerned with the moon in all her phases, with dreams, birth and death, with the hidden aspects of life that we nurture in the warm darkness of our minds as a woman nurtures the unborn child. In the teachings of the Qabalah Yesod is also called 'The Foundation'. This gives a feeling of strength, and indeed the angels of Yesod are named 'The Cherubim' or 'The Strong Ones'. A foundation must be strong in order to uphold that which is placed over it. This ritual is designed to bring about the realization of the inner strength and power that a true magical mating can evoke. Yesod is also the gateway to the Land of Dreams, Magic and the Dark Wood of Enchantment. This book will offer you many ways to change your life and the way you live your life. But to make those changes you must first pass through the Gate of Wonder into the Land of Dreams.

The Moon Goddess has three faces, as most of you reading this will know. They are the Maiden, the Wife, and the Wise Woman, sometimes called the Hag or Crone. A woman holds all three within herself from birth, when they are potential. Each comes to the fore and manifests at the moment ordained, bringing their gifts and their sorrows, til death, and as the Wise Woman closes her eyes for the last time, the Maiden and the Wife are still held within, fulfilled at last.

In the Rite of Pan, the man was the 'hunter' and the woman the 'prey' in the eternal chase that has little to do with which sex is dominant, and everything to do with the readying and stimulation of the physical body for mating. When that last bit is understood you can forget the argument of who is top dog and concentrate on equality of beingness. Man is strong within the earth sphere, woman is equally strong in the sphere above that. This can be seen in the Tarot Trump of The Lovers (see Fig 6). Here the man is unable to communicate with the angelic level as clearly as the woman, so looks to her for help. She looks up to receive the angelic communication which she will then pass across to her partner.

In the Ritual of the Moon Cup the woman is 'the summoner' and the man is 'the summoned'. She is the Moon's Daughter, her representative on earth; he is the Lord of the Forest who pays homage to the moon for his domain. The term 'forest lord' can be equated with Herne the Hunter, the Horned Lord with his antlered crown, the Leader of the Wild Hunt, etc. Lord he may be of the wild places of the earth, but to keep them he must acknowledge his lunar mistress, for it is by her light that he hunts, and the price is his seed, given to the moon, which she uses to pass from the slender crescent of the new moon to the burgeoning roundness of the full moon.[1]

The moon has always been the prime symbol of woman, ruling her monthly cycle as well as the seas and oceans of the world. In the new crescent, the full moon and the waning moon she shows again the three faces of the Goddess that are reflected in every human woman. Her names are many: Artemis, Diana, Selene, Cynthia, Celemon, Aradia, Isis, Tanith, Hecate and others. She governs growth in all things: on the physical level she rules the growth from seedling to babe, and on the inner level she brings to birth her moonchildren – ideas, thoughts, and energies that either stay with her as unresolved dreams or descend to become realities in the form of paintings, poems, music and all forms of creativity. The unknown prehistoric artist who drew 'The Dancing Sorcerer' owed his skill as much to the ability to moondream his subject as to the flexibility of his hand and fingers.

The moon is the giver of inspiration and the ability to make dreams come true and her daughter, woman, shares this ability. The saying that 'behind every great man there is a strong woman' is more than just an old wives' tale. While women are more than capable of becoming great leaders in their own right, there are many who prefer to help their partner make either his own dream or their shared dreams come true. Either way woman is the inspiration of man, either as a physical being or in the form of the feminine Muse. She is the sustainer, the nurturer, and as the

[1] The names of the 12 full moons are given in the Dusty Millar Lunar Calendar.

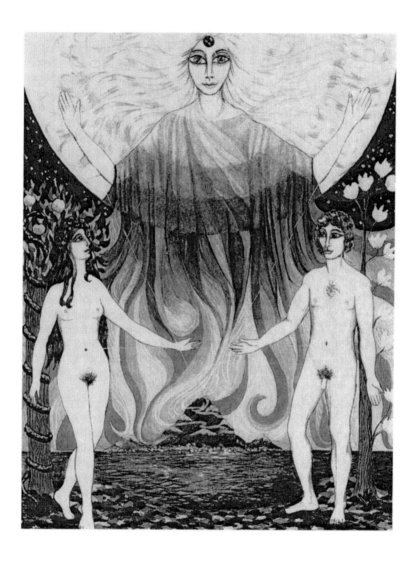

*Figure 6:* The Lovers *(Jo Gill, from The Servants of the Light Tarot)*

sphere of Binah, one of the great supernals of the Tree of Life, she is understanding. When you take that word apart you will find it holds the same meaning as 'the Foundation' – that which stands beneath and lends its strength to that which is above.

In the Tarot Trump of The Moon we see depicted the strange water creature that crawls out of the pool, symbolizing the emergence of life from the oceans of pre-history. The effect of the moon on those far off seas was the same as it is today, a rocking motion as the tide flows in and out, a motion that acted as a mother's arms act around a human baby, rocking it, soothing it, comforting the pains of growth. In the same way a woman comforts modern man with her presence in his life, and in her arms he may find the comfort of the almost forgotten Moon Mother to whom ancient man looked for comfort and guidance.

This ritual is an outdoor one, though it can be worked inside. Nevertheless if it is in any way possible it must be done out of doors. The very heart of it needs the feeling of freedom and space. If there is nowhere near that is private and quiet and *safe*, I suggest you ask a friend or even a sympathetic relative for the use of their garden – always providing you can rely on their discretion to leave you alone. If you really want to do the ritual you will find a way to do it, however I cannot over-emphasize the need for safety and privacy. There are not many places where you can be sure of those two essentials. It is time some private landowners with suitable woodlands and sympathy towards the pagan need for seclusion and privacy offered to loan or even hire for a modest sum the use of their land to those who can provide references to their reliability and trustworthiness. There is a great need in people to worship under the sky as their ancestors did long ago, and need should be met.

Ideally your location for this ritual should offer tree cover dense enough to light a small fire so that if the ritual is worked during the colder months you will at least have some warmth. It should also offer a clear pathway so that the one who is summoned may see and approach the sacred circle and the priestess who awaits him. If you light a fire, be careful to see that it is contained and cannot get out of hand. Keep a blanket handy to smother any flames that may catch dry wood alight. Work magic outdoors by all means, but *make sure you act in a responsible manner towards the environment*.

The rite itself revolves around the communion between the moon and her daughter, the priestess, and the preparation and casting of the circle. The summoning of the Lord of the Forest and his approach to the circle is the second part of the rite, and as he cannot enter without permission, he must persuade the priestess to allow it. Once within the circle he comes under the power of the moon, is bound to her service and must pay homage to her priestess. The inner meaning of the ritual is centred around and consecrated by the sexual fluids of the male and female. When mixed together they form a potent power element that has been known and used in the Middle and Far East for more than a thousand years. It is only in the West, where the art and practice of sex both for pleasure and as a means of worship has been denounced as a perversity and a sin, that ignorance rules supreme.

The preparations begin as always a week before the actual rite, and the same rules of celibacy for that week will apply as before (sorry about that!) Always hold in mind that for any kind of sex to be truly fulfilling the two people concerned must be in harmony. Where the sex is part of a magical ceremony they must mesh physically, emotionally, mentally and spiritually, and to achieve this the physical body must be tuned like a musical instrument through all its levels. There is no way sexual magic can be practised safely unless both partners know each other well and have worked together for a long time. This kind of work is not for the high priest/priestess and the latest neophyte, so be warned.

Now we move on to the exercises for this particular ritual. I will give those for the woman first.

On first waking turn on to your back and stretch each leg right down to the toes. Now stretch the arms, just as you did with the first ritual. Move slowly, do not rush things. Get up and reach up over your head and stretch your spine, allow your body to flop over and down so that your head, arms and hands hang down limply in front of you and just brush the floor with your fingertips if you can. Now curve the spine and come up slowly, letting each vertebra settle into place.

If you look at Fig 7 you will see that there are two energy lines encompassing the body. Both start in the same place, the base chakra or perineum. These energy lines were discovered hundreds of years ago by the Masters of Tao. They also found that the energy these lines carry, although ending at separate places, can be joined to complete a circuit of power that the body can use to strengthen, heal and energize the cells and the major organs of the body.

The broken line flows from its source at the perineum up the front of the body, touching the intestines, the bowels, the uterus, heart and lungs. It ends at the tip of the tongue. The dotted line flows up the spine into and through the brain and down to the roof of the mouth. The simple action of touching the tongue to the roof of the mouth (see Fig 8) links both energy lines together and allows the flow to circulate right around the body.

The first exercise consists of sitting on a chair with the spine upright. Draw the chin in and down just a little, relax the

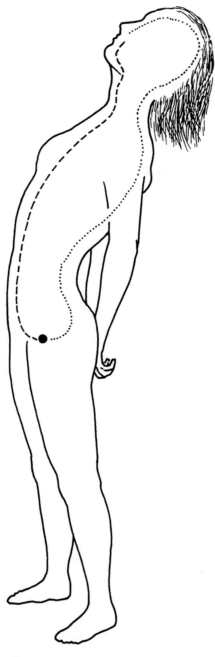

*Figure 7*: Energy lines

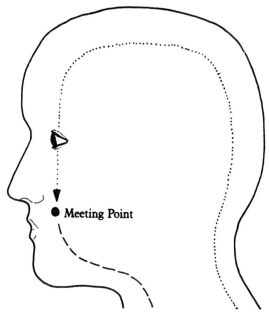

*Figure 8:* Linking the energy lines

shoulders, touch the tongue to the roof of the mouth and breathe in deeply, visualizing the energy flowing like twin flashes of light emanating from the centre point, one travelling up the spine, the other up the front of the body, and uniting where the tongue meets the roof of the mouth. Now let the tongue fall away and gently blow the air out through pursed lips. Do this at least six times, more if you have the time. The energy thus accumulated will be stored in the body for use when needed. (If you wear dentures remove them, for the tongue *must* touch the actual roof of the mouth.)

The second exercise for the woman is as above, but this time breathe more slowly and allow the energy to 'light up' the organs and the vertebrae as it passes through them. To seal the energy in, press two fingers to the top of the head and two fingers to the perineum for a count of five. Do four to five breaths and then seal the energy. This concludes the woman's morning exercises.

The exercises for the man are as follows. Kneel on the floor with the knees about nine or ten inches apart but with the feet touching behind the body. You might like to use one of the small wooden seats available for those who cannot sit easily in this position. Most esoteric or health food shops have them in stock. Place the hands on the thighs at right angles, which will cause the elbows to jut out to the side. Keep the spine erect and look straight ahead. Take in just half the usual amount of air and retain it, but without locking the throat. Keep the throat open as a singer does before using the air to sing a note. Now follow the same instructions as for the first set of female exercises. The reason for the different position is to allow the scrotum more freedom, as constriction of this part of the body during the exercises will impede the vital flow of energy it needs.

The second exercise for the man has been practised in the Far East for over a thousand years and is still practised today. Translated from the original language its Chinese title means 'the Dance of the Testicles'. There are some variations that you may come across in your reading but all look for the same result, an increase of energy flow throughout the whole body.

Sit on the edge of a straight-backed chair with feet flat on the floor but not together. The room should be comfortably warm and the clothing, if any, must be loose. Focus the inner attention on a point between the two testicles. Inhale slowly and draw them up, hold the breath for a count of four, then breathe out and lower the testicles again. This is the first part of the exercise. Use your imagination to 'see' the energy of the breath filling up the testes with its force. Each breath leaves a little more energy there until you can feel that whole area filled with it.

It is important that you keep both the penis and the anus as relaxed as possible. Continue as before but now draw the energy further, as far as the perineum, always making sure that you draw the testicles up with the in breath and let them down with the out breath. At first you may notice no movement, or very little, but with perseverance you will soon begin to see actual movement within the scrotum sac.

The evening exercises are done by both the man and woman together and are very simple as well as pleasurable.

If you are not using the oil specially created for these rituals by Golden Lotus, then I would suggest oil of cedar or sandalwood for the man and perhaps oil of juniper for the woman in these exercises.[2] Remember that all essential oils are highly concentrated and you will need a carrier oil such as sweet almond or plain olive oil for the massage. Never use a pure essential oil directly on to the skin, especially around the genitals as it can be far too strong for the delicate skin in that area and may cause severe irritation. Use three to four drops of the essential oil to a bottle of carrier oil.

After your evening shower or bath, wrap yourselves in warmed bath towels, and make a nest of pillows against the bedhead so

[2] Oils of high quality may be obtained from Margaret Bruce direct, see the address at the back of book, or from reliable esoteric stockists.

that whoever goes first may lie back and fully relax. The other person sits on the bed and takes their partner's right foot in their lap with a small towel or cloth beneath it, pours a small amount of oil into the hands and begins to massage the foot. There are an amazing number of nerve endings in the hands and feet and yet most lovers pay little or no attention to them during their love play. Vary your touch from light stroking through to very firm kneading and keep using small quantities of oil to keep the hands sliding over the skin. Change to the left foot and repeat the process, then the right hand and finally the left hand. Allow a minimum of 15 minutes for the complete massage, but not more than 20, or your partner will fall asleep before you have had your turn. Change places and oils and repeat the process.

This is not all there is to the exercise, which utilizes four of the five senses: sight (of your partner), touch and smell from the massage and the oil, and lastly the sense of hearing. (If you wish to add the fifth sense to the exercise, have a glass of your favourite wine nearby to sip.) The sensual effect is completed by the spoken word, the praise of the God in the man and the Goddess in the woman. This should preferably be learned by heart, but may be written out, placed nearby and read out. However, done in this way it loses 90 per cent of its power to arouse the senses.

First the invocation to the Goddess, spoken by the man to the woman:

> Thou art the White One, Daughter of the Night, my love and my delight. In thee lies all my happiness, my power, and my strength. Within the arms of the Moon's Daughter I take my rest and offer all that is within myself to thee and to the Great Mother that rules us both. I come from the depths of the forest, the Leader of the Wild Hunt. No man may stand against me. Lord of all warriors am I, yet with thee I am the gentle unicorn laying my magical horn in thy lap. These feet may wind me round with dancing steps, these hands may caress or command me, for I am the guardian of she who belongs to no other being but herself, the maid, the virgin, the one attained yet ever unattainable. Thou art the moon's sweet daughter, my love and my delight, and I am he who shall be thy love. Shine forth from this moment, my lady moon, that in joining with your daughter I shall join with all three, the maid, the wife, and the wisest of all, the moon's dark self. Prepare thyself for me when the time shall come and my horn shall lie in thy lap in homage to all womanhood.

This should be spoken with feeling and a sense of awe.

The woman's invocation:

> Hail to thee, Lord of the Forest, hail to thee, the horned, crowned rider of the night sky. From the depths of the wood I shall call thee to my side when the time be right, and in my arms thou shalt find sleep and forgetfulness of all but the old ways. Thou art strong of body and

of spirit. Together we shall ride the night winds. Herne, Cernunnos, Kernan, Gwynn ap Nudd, many are thy names. I see only you, my love and my lord. Let me know thy touch and the sweetness of thy mouth. The power and the grace of thee shall wrap me around with fire and deep within the sacred centre of my womanhood I will welcome thee as king to my queen, air to my fire, water to my earth. To the fountain of thy force I shall be the waiting pool, to the upstanding corn I shall be the scythe, to the athame I shall be the chalice. I shall call the wild one from within thee to the appointed place at the appointed time.

These are not just pretty speeches, they are potent invocations to archetypes that are older than humanity, so do them justice.

Apart from the specially made oils mentioned you will need an incense strong enough to be used outside. A good mixture would be frankincense, sandalwood and a little camphor, or of course you can use the incense made specially for this ritual. Music is not always appropriate in an outside setting unless you are sure of absolute privacy, but if you have to conduct the ritual inside and you would like music, then try some of the New Age tapes that feature environmental music with nature sounds such as rainfall and running water within the musical structure.

To augment the invocations provided you might like to select some of Shakespeare's sonnets to read out. They are undoubtedly some of the finest love lyrics ever written. If you are among those who feel foolish speaking Shakespearean verse (in which case High Magic is not going to be easy for you with its long and sonorous invocations), then try speaking in your own words, always providing they are a little more magical than 'Are you ready yet?'

Meditation on suitable symbols should be included in your daily routine, either with the morning exercises or in the evening. These symbols would include a white hart, a twelve-tined stag, a chalice with a crescent moon pouring water into it, a dolmen on a sacred mound under a full moon, a unicorn and a single pearl.

The same rules apply to this ritual as to the first: privacy, no telephone, arrange your time so that the afternoon is free for preparations. Choose a time when the moon is new; this is not a ritual for a waning moon.

The things you will need for an outdoor ritual will differ slightly from those needed for an indoor one. For outdoors you will need two lanterns, the kind that use candles rather than paraffin; a groundsheet and a thick blanket to go over it; a chalice and a bottle of red wine; oil for the anointing; a basket of fruit and almond or coconut cakes (both can be ascribed to the moon); a small basket of rice or corn kernels; salt and water already consecrated and mixed together; some mixed herbs and spices and fragrant leaves and flower heads. If you have a cauldron then use it as a fire pit and incense burner combined and put a thick layer of sand in the bottom, placing the charcoal on top, then you can burn the incense safely. If you are going to use music then you will need a small cassette player and the tapes you have chosen. The Daughter of the Moon should wear a robe that opens right down the front in dark blue, silver or white, and sandals, with her hair loose and crowned with a garland of leaves and whatever white flowers are in season. She will also need either a short sword or a moon-shaped sickle. Beneath the robe is a girdle/belt of ivy that goes around the waist and between the thighs and attaches to the belt at the back. The ivy should be young and easily snapped – too old and tough and your priestess might just as well be wearing a medieval chastity belt! A wood-cloak will keep off any chill and has the added advantage of making its wearer almost invisible against the trees at night.[3]

The Lord of the Forest will need a belt to carry the athame; a wood-cloak; sandals or soft shoes; a small gift for the Moon's Daughter which should not be seen by her until its giving, if it is possible to find one; a small hunting horn; and lastly a small silver coin. If he feels 'unsafe' wearing nothing beneath his cloak the man may wear a pair of old jeans, but they must be perfectly clean (beneath the jeans there should only be bare flesh, so the Moon Priestess should be extremely careful when handling the zip!)

If the rite is taking place indoors then you must clear a space for it. Remove as much furniture as possible and clean the floor thoroughly. Cover it with one or two clean sheets and make this your sacred area. Spread the blanket in the middle and instead of the lanterns use candles set around the room, but make sure they cannot be overturned by accident. The room should be warm enough to be comfortable and all that you need should be close to hand.

---

[3] A wood-cloak is a cape of any thick warm material lined with soft cotton and coming down to the top of the heel. It has a deep hood that can be pulled forward completely, hiding the face. The outer material is either black, dark green, russet brown or dark blue with a lining of the same colour. With no shiny buttons or clasps to flash in the moon or lantern light it is the perfect garment for working out of doors. In the Traditional Craft it is usually worn with nothing beneath, providing the weather plays fair.

# The Ritual of the Moon Cup

## Place on the Tree = Yesod. Keynotes = Magic, Dreams and Inner Strength.

*The ritual assumes you will be working outside. If this is not possible use the suggestions above for an indoor rite.*

*The Moon's Daughter goes ahead to prepare the sacred place, which should be positioned to catch as much moonlight as possible. First mark out a large circle with either the sword or the sickle, making it large enough to accommodate the action of the ritual. Inside this circle lay out the groundsheet so that it covers the central area. This ritual needs no direction points other than the point of moonrise, which is taken as the altar point of the circle. Here you can lay down a small white cloth and place on it the chalice with the opened wine nearby, the three baskets of fruit and cakes, rice/corn kernels and herbs, spices and fragrant leaves, also the salt and water and oils.*

*Opposite is placed the cauldron, prepared with a base of sand topped with fresh charcoal, together with the incense and matches. The two lanterns can be placed either within the circle or, if you prefer, can be hung from the trees. The blanket is folded and placed to one side. When all is in place the sacring of the circle may begin. The incense is lit and then the priestess takes the salt and water and following the circle round she casts drops of the hallowed mixture on the earth to cleanse the whole area*

*Priestess:* With the tears of my mother the moon and the sweat of my sister the earth, I cleanse this place of all impurity and make it sacred for the rite.

*She returns to the starting point, picks up the basket of rice/corn and repeats the circling.*

With this gift of my sister the earth, I feed the younger brethren and ask them to share with us the joys of this night's work.

*She replaces the basket, goes to collect the cauldron and replenishes the incense, then takes it around the circle to the starting point at its original place and sets it down.*

With the fire of the earth's inner heart I ward this place of sacred rite, with the fire of my own inner heart I set it about with symbols of protection, with burning herbs I invoke the spirits of tree and bush, flower and bud, to lend their power to this night's work, with the rising of incense I invoke the spirits of the air to build about us a bower of dreams.

*She takes the basket of herbs and spices to scatter over the centre of the circle.*

Moon, my mother, earth, my sister, be with me tonight in body, in heart, in mind, in spirit. Guide the Hunter of the Forest to this sacred bower that we may join as thou hast ordained for the joy of man and woman since the beginning of time. In that joining let all about us be blessed as we shall be blessed. Make me, O Moon Mother, thine own sweet self, that in his worship of thee I may also be worshipped as woman, symbolic of all my sisters. Let all things, seen and unseen, rejoice in the filling of the moon cup.

*She stands before the cauldron, raises her arms to the moon and bows three times. She continues, loudly:*

In the name of the moon, my mother, I call thee, Hunter of the Forest, I call thee by the moon's sacred light, I call thee by oak and thorn and by sacred rowan, by red berry and white flower, I call thee by the gentle doe and the twelve-tined stag, by white dove and grey hawk. I call thee by the leaping salmon and silver trout, by pink lip and bright eye, by the soft breast and the shadowed thigh. From the high hill and the dark wood, from lea and field, from home and hearth I summon thee to the sacred circle to mate with the Moon's Daughter. Answer, answer, answer.

*The Hunter allows a full two minutes to pass then either winds the horn or sends his call of 'Ah-hi-ee' on three ascending notes ringing through the wood. He then moves a quarter circle, waits a minute and repeats the call. He does this until a full circle has been completed. He waits another minute and then steps into view but beyond the circle.*

*Hunter:* I greet thee, Daughter of the Moon, the summons reached me as I rode the night path and I have left the Wild Hunt to attend thee. What is the reason for the call?

*Priestess:* I have called thee to the circle cast in the ancient ways that the greatest rite of all may be celebrated. The moon cup must be filled and I have need of thy strength and thy manhood. Is it thy will to follow the ancient law?

*Hunter:* My strength is needed for the Hunt. If I give it to you who will ride the night path? Who will protect the small wild things and the lost spirits that call for comfort?

*Priestess:* The Moon Mother will guide the Hunt and stand guard in your place. Come to me, Hunter of the Night, come and pay homage as men have done since the moon first walked the heavens when the earth was young. I stand in lieu of all womankind, in mating with me you shall mate with them and in the love death shall you be reborn.

*Hunter:* The circle is closed against me, how may I enter and claim the Moon's Daughter? What key unlocks the gate?

*Priestess:* By the payment of a silver coin to the earth, my sister, a token that will lift the wards, by the cutting of the circle with the knife, a token to the spirits that you respect their powers, by the giving of a gift, a token to the Moon's Daughter to woo her smile.

*The Hunter presses a silver coin deep into the earth beneath the cauldron, then with the athame he cuts through the circle and steps*

*through, drawing the knife across the cut immediately afterwards. He
then comes to stand before the priestess and bows and offers her the little
gift. This she places by the chalice and turns to the Hunter.*

*Priestess:* Not so easily am I won. First answer me this: I am as
young as the newborn lamb and as old as a man's last breath, my
head and feet are cold but my heart holds fire, my womb is never
empty but no man can hold me in his arms: what is my name?

*Hunter:* Your name is Gaia, the earth. I win, priestess!

*Priestess:* I touch the earth but never set foot upon it, I walk
upon the sea yet my feet are never wet, I have 12 names but no
mother or father: who am I?

*Hunter:* You are the moon. I am near to my prize.

*Priestess:* We were born at the same birth, yet we can never
touch, we look alike yet must remain each other's opposite, we
can never part, never speak and must die together: what is my
nature?

*Hunter:* You are your own reflection. Now I claim thee, my
summoner, my life and my death.

*Priestess:* Hunter, you have passed my test. The way is open to
you. Draw near and join me in invoking the great lunar mother,
for without her consent no joining of man and woman is valid.

*They join hands and turn to face the moon and bow three times. The
priestess takes the chalice and holds it up to the moon.*

*Priestess:* Mother and Goddess, lightgiver amid darkness, fill this
chalice with thy radiance and power, fill it with the ecstasy that
comes when two that are separate and different become one and
the same. I am the chalice of womanhood, fill me also with these
things. Descend into me, Great Mother, and let the gift of love be
our gift to thee. So mote it be this moonfilled night.

*She turns to the Hunter with the chalice. He draws the athame and
holds it high, then slowly brings is down until it enters the chalice.*

*Hunter:* I have answered the summons of the Moon's Daughter.
Only through her eyes may I see the hidden things of the spirit.
Show me the way to the Land of the Ever-becoming. Guide me
between the ivory hills that rise up, star-tipped, to greet me. Open
to me the sacred doorway that lies hidden behind the Forest of
Dreams.

*Priestess:* The key lies in the chalice of the moon and the wine it
will contain. Together the Moon's Daughter and Lord of the Forest
will prepare the earth for this coming moon. Come, my lord and
love, and I will anoint thee with oil.

*The priestess folds back the wood-cloak and if necessary removes any
other clothing from the Hunter. With the oil she anoints the forehead,
throat, breastbone, navel, the head of the phallus, the knees and the arch
of the foot, using the symbol of the crescent moon and kissing each place
before using the oil.*

*Priestess:* Moon to Hunter, thus do I pass to thee my powers in the inner world.

*The Hunter folds back the cloak of the priestess and loosens her gown, opening it completely. Taking the oil he anoints the forehead, throat, each breast, the womb, the labia, the knees and the arch of the foot, kissing each place before using the oil as before.*

*Hunter:* Hunter to Moon, thus do I pass to thee my powers within the forest and the Wild Hunt. One more key must I have from thee, Daughter of the Moon, before the rite can come to power.

*He kneels before her, hands on her hips, forehead resting on her belly.*

*Hunter:* Will you yield to me the right to cut the sacred kestos?[4]

*Priestess:* For this night alone, I yield to thee that right.

*The Hunter draws his athame and cuts through the ivy, freeing her completely. He stands, raises the athame high.*

*Hunter:* Hail to thee, Moon Mother, the last key has been given freely and accepted humbly.

*The Hunter brings the folded blanket, spreads it for his priestess and removes her cloak. She lies down and the Hunter brings his cloak over them both. It is important to take your time and allow the passion of moon and forest to rise to its fullest extent before the mating begins.*

*Priestess:* Lord of the Forest, the moon path lies open to thee and the gateway to the Hidden Land of Dreams yields its secrets, for they are mine alone to give or withhold.

*She opens her thighs and holds up her arms to enfold him.*

*Hunter:* Daughter of the Moon, the victory is yours and I pass through the gate into the Cave of Stars.

*Penetration should be effected slowly and with care, and only when fully joined may the mating begin. The priestess holds the crescent symbol in her mind, seeing it as the chalice. The Hunter holds the symbol of the athame or the lightning flash in his thoughts and the two must be visualized together, with one filling the other, superimposed on the night sky as the sexual climax occurs. The sensuality of the moment is offered up to the Moon Mother for Her purpose of revitalizing Nature.*

*The Hunter withdraws and both kneel with the chalice held in the hands of the priestess. The mingled fluids of the ritual mating are sparingly used to anoint the inside of the chalice which is then filled with wine. Hunter and priestess stand and share a sip of the wine together then, moving together, they circle the sacred place and cast drops of the moon wine onto the earth.*

*Priestess:* Wine of the moon, drawn from the earth and empowered by woman's spirit and man's strength, fill the earth with joy, love and peace.

---

[4] The kestos is the belt of chastity worn by the ancient priestesses of certain temples. Its removal by a man, unless a chosen priest, was forbidden.

*Hunter:* We give what has been drawn from us freely and with knowingness and power.

*Priestess:* Earth and heaven, joined and enriched by moon and forest, receive our blessing.

*Hunter:* In giving we shall also receive and be made holy.

*Priestess:* Moon Mother, take our offering and with it fill the earth with life.

*Hunter:* Earth sister, be one with us in our joy this night.

*Any wine left in the chalice is drunk, the wood-cloaks put on and Hunter and Priestess face each other.*

*Priestess:* Hunter, Lord of the Forest, I bless thee in the name of the Moon Mother for thy gift of seed this night. For thy gentleness I thank thee, for the sweetness of thy love I thank thee. I set thee free now to follow the way of the wild hunt. I gift thee with a kiss.

*She kisses him.*

*Hunter:* Lady and priestess, Daughter of the Moon, earth's sister, to thee my homage and my love. For the precious gift of thy body I bless thee, for what we have shared I thank thee, in service I kneel to thee.

*He kneels and kisses her hand, then leaves the circle for the darkness of the forest. The priestess may now offer her own prayer if she desires. She gathers all that has been used together and scatters any rice, herbs, salt and water that is left over the earth in blessing. The man and woman now depart.*

# The Pathworking

A new moon rides high in a clear sky, and a cool wind blows the trees into a frenzy. Before us lies a dark forest and from it comes the chilling howl of a wolf. A cold prickle of apprehension raises the hair on the back of our necks and we turn to see a band of horsemen come riding over the hill behind us. Their clothes are varied as if they have been drawn from many different times in the earth's history, and indeed they have, for this is the Wild Hunt. To its brotherhood are drawn ancient warriors and chieftains, the lost and the tormented and those unwilling to conform. Yet they are not damned souls, they ride under the leadership of the Lord of the Forest, Herne the Hunter, the antler-crowned, the lover of the Moon's Daughter.

Herne guides and disciplines the men who ride with him and through their work of protecting those who have need of them, they may one day leave the Hunt and be reborn. Until then they ride the dark nights hunting those who serve the Lord of the Dark

Face. They ride at full gallop but no sound is heard from their headlong rush, for the hooves of their mounts do not quite touch the earth. Weapons gleam in the dim light and the jingle of the harness is the only sound we can hear . . .

Then from the forest comes a song, a woman's voice as silver as the moon, delicate and sweet. The melody rises and falls and weaves patterns that enchain the emotions, it calls and summons the one for whom it is meant.

We see the Hunt wheel and its leader's horse rears up onto its back legs, but the rider sits firm. He turns to the forest and we see a strong face with dark brows shadowing clear grey eyes. His dark hair flows to his shoulders and the sweep of the antlers that crown his head add to his majesty of bearing. The call comes again and he looks up to the crescent moon and smiles. The men around him laugh and seem to joke among themselves. For a moment he is silent, then he beckons to one of the warriors and speaks with him. The man bows his head and gathers the Hunt about him, and in a few moments they are heading towards the north star, leaving Herne alone.

He sits looking towards the forest for a while, then for a third time the silver song is heard and he lifts his horn to his lips and answers it and rides towards the trees and his love.

Like wraiths we drift behind him and see him ride into the darkness, bending in the saddle to avoid the small branches tangling with his antlers. He follows no path yet seems to know exactly where the singer is hiding. We follow unseen, twisting and turning, until we see ahead of us the glow of a fire. Herne dismounts and leaves his horse to go on foot.

In a clearing stands a young woman with a clear pale complexion and dark hair that flows to her knees. Her hair is her only covering and through it we can see glimpses of the loveliness beneath. Forming a large circle around her is a ring of white flame that dances and curls yet does not burn the grass. It is the cold moonfire that guards and protects the Moon's Daughter.

She holds out her arms to her love and he draws his sword and with it cuts through the flame which bends and allows him entry, but springs up again behind him. Their meeting is that of lovers long a part of each other's existence. Herne swings his cloak from his shoulders and spreads it on the ground to make a bed for his lady, and from within his tunic he brings a gift for her, a rope of pearls that match her skin and take their glow from her smile.

Without his rough woven tunic and breeches the Leader of the Wild Hunt is seen to be a fitting mate for the beauty of the Moon Priestess. She winds her hair about him, making him a willing prisoner, and draws him down to lie in her arms. There is no shame in their mating, only joy and beauty; we feel no shame to watch them for we know that this is more than man and woman, more than Herne and priestess, it is the archetypal union of heaven and earth, moon and forest, mortal and immortal. Herne lifts his head and cries out, a sound that goes ringing through the forest and far beyond, then the antlers drop and he rests his head on her breast, her arms holding him closely to her heart.

We leave them and return to the hill where the Hunt has returned and waits quietly for their leader to rejoin them. Sometimes when the Moon's Daughter mates with the Leader of the Wild Hunt, they offer their joy in each other to the Gods and in return the Gods choose one of the Hunt to be reborn on earth with all that has gone before forgiven him.

Suddenly one of the huntsmen raises his head. There is a look of joy and wonder on his face and it is clear to his companions that his time of release is near. The others draw back as he dismounts, goes to the very top of the hill and stands with his arms raised. A radiance gathers about him, increasing in intensity until we can no longer see him, then it is gone and the top of the hill is empty.

From the forest Herne comes riding. When he reaches the hill the Hunt regroups about him and with one last look back to the forest he leads them away. We watch as they ride off, their horses gradually mounting up into the night sky and wheeling at full gallop towards the Milky Way. Behind us the forest is still and silent, and the Moon's Daughter sleeps wrapped in the Hunter's cloak, wearing a rope of pearls.

# Ritual 3

# THE DANCE OF LOVE

## The Programme

Before you attempt this ritual it might be of help if first you were to read some of the Hindu legends and try to grasp the concept of Mother India's many Gods and Goddesses. You will find as you go on through the rituals that they are arranged so as to emphasize the masculine and feminine powers alternately, with some of them acting as balancing rituals where both sexes have an equal part to play. These balancing rituals occur in the spheres of Tiphereth and Kether, and in the 'un-named' ritual of Da'ath.

The ritual pertaining to the sphere of Hod is complex and difficult to remember, but it *must* be committed to memory: to keep looking at a script would completely destroy the whole atmosphere and might conceivably cause physical repercussions. These would almost certainly mean problems with the sexual energies, especially maintaining an erection in the male partner, and a loss of sexual desire over a period of time for either partner. Always remember that where these rituals are concerned you are dealing with advanced powers and failure to get things right can result in dysfunction of the sexual natures.

It is time perhaps to issue another warning. Remember this book is for those who have been practising the art of magic for a considerable time, *not* for the beginners, the power trippers, the foolish and the profane. What you are being taught to deal with is the great primary power of the universe, the creative force. This force makes galaxies out of star matter, but it also destroys them when they go wrong. Knowing that, think what it can do to you if it is mishandled. Going nova in your bedroom is not part of my plan for the readers of this book!

This third ritual is based on the Hindu triune of Brahma the Creator, Vishnu the Protector and Shiva the Destroyer, together with the Goddesses or Shaktis Saraswati, Laxshmi and Kali. The male symbol is the lingam or phallus, the female symbol is the yoni or vagina, and there are many representations of both of them throughout Indian mythology.

The Hindu pantheon is very complicated and each God and Goddess may have many variations on their name. Briefly, Brahma, Vishnu and Shiva can be seen as birth, life, and death or transcendence. Each God/Shakta is part of and inseparable from the Shakti or Goddess that is his female self. In just the same way each Goddess is part of and inseparable from the God that is her male self. So there is really a multiple God form that has three male and three female aspects. Brahma and Saraswati are the creative pair, the parents, the patrons of the arts. Vishnu and Laxshmi are the preservers of life, the givers of prosperity and fortune. Shiva and Kali are the Death Gods, the givers of transcendental experience. Let's take a closer look at each pair.

The Upanishads say of Brahma that he is the creator of all things – from him came space, air, fire, water and earth. His symbol is a golden egg. Saraswati is the patroness of the 64 arts, foremost of which is the art of love. Her symbol is the seven-stringed vina, a musical instrument said to be evocative of a woman's body in shape. The seven strings symbolize the seven rays of creation that are echoed all through nature in the colours of the rainbow, in the musical scale (where the eighth note is a higher form of the first), and in the seven centres of the subtle body. Both Brahma and Saraswati are visualized as being golden in body colour and radiating golden light. In the art of Tantra when a man and a woman identify with them they become the archetypal male and female.

Vishnu is the God who maintains the universe so that life may evolve in all its myriad forms. He cares for and protects that life. His body colour is blue and it is held that he manifests on the earth in many different forms or avatars. His symbols are the conch shell and the discus. Laxshmi, his Shakti, is analogous to Aphrodite in many ways. Said to be more beautiful than the rising sun, she is sensuality itself. She is either red or white in colour and holds a lotus flower as her emblem. When identification with these God forms is achieved the art of love becomes perfected in all its forms.

Shiva is transcendent life, pure conscious thought, the conqueror of the state of death. His colour is white and his symbol is the trident. Kali is the liberator, the four-armed Goddess, the great night of time. Her colour is black and her main symbol is the sword. She is usually pictured standing or squatting in sexual union on the body of Shiva holding in her upper left arm the sword and in her lower left a severed head. The two arms on the opposite side have hands that make gestures of protectiveness and blessing respectively. To achieve full identification with these supreme beings can take many years of practice and effort, and you will not be able to do this without going through the many levels of Tantra under the guidance of an adept of this particular path. However you may be able to gain an insight into the power and transcendental energy of the Shakta and Shakti through the following ritual.

During the time in which the rite is accomplished you will become each divine couple in turn, for the intention of the ritual is to identify with them in a cosmic cycle taking the couple from creation, through life and into and beyond the transmutation of death. This is achieved through an integrated process of music, dance, poetry, sexual union and visualization. Each stage will require its own mood, position, inner images and symbols. To bring all this together in one ritual will require a lot of study, effort and skill. As I have already said, this is a difficult and complex ritual but I have also pointed out that this is a book for advanced ritualists. You may ask what it is that will make this so difficult, so let me tell you.

1) The ritual takes place gradually over the whole day, beginning at sunrise with the first mating in honour of Brahma and Saraswati. At noon it continues with the one for Vishnu and Laxshmi, and ends at sunset with the ritual for Shiva and Kali.

2) Three ejaculations in one day, albeit staggered (probably the wrong word!) over 12 hours, may enable the male partner to give a very good imitation indeed of Shiva as the 'dead' God form over which Kali dances out the transformation of his substance.

3) You will need to keep the power flowing and hold on to the God forms all through those 12 hours, with a gradual transformation from one to the other at noon and again at sunset.

My suggestion is that you take a whole weekend for this ritual, starting your preparations on the Friday night, and using the Sunday to recover.

The morning exercises for the woman are as follows. First warm up your muscles by swinging your arms from side to side, slowly at first and working up to a brisk swing. Now bend from the waist and catch hold of each leg in turn just behind the knee and gently bring the head in as far as you can. *Do not force in any way.* Repeat with the other side. Now continue with the rest of the exercises. Have a straight-backed chair close by. Fold a small towel in half and sit on it with the body held erect but not stiffly. Let the

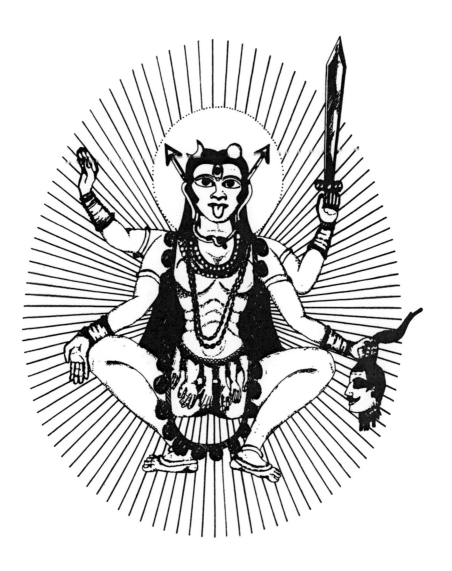

*Figure 9:* Kali

shoulders relax. Bring the knees up and place the soles of the feet together. Hold them in this position with your hands and allow the knees to fall outwards as far as is comfortable for you. Making sure that the feet are firmly pressed together, place hands on the thighs and alternately tense and relax the thigh muscles. Do this 10 times, then press the soles of the feet together as hard as you can and relax. Do this 10 times as well. Then, very gently, with your hands on your knees, press the knees towards the ground – but very very gently, you do not want to pull the muscles. The aim is to gradually loosen the muscles until the knees can fall outwards and touch, or almost touch, the ground. Remember this exercise is for the woman only.

Now place – or get your partner to place – a chair between your thighs in such a way as to allow you, with your knees bent and slightly raised, to hook your legs around the legs of the chair. Use your heels to hold the chair securely. Now with the perineum as flat to the floor as you can get it, tighten and relax the thighs 10 times. Now repeat the exercise but at the same time tighten and *hold* both the thigh muscles and the vaginal muscles for a count of five. Relax. Do this five times on the first day and add two each successive day.

For the male partner the day will start with the second exercise from the last ritual. This is to be done every day. Added to that is the following. Sit crossed-legged on the floor with the body well centred and a small towel folded beneath you to act as a support. Keep the spine erect but supple, place another small towel under the crossed feet to raise and support them. Fold your hands one over the other, palms up, and get your partner to place several heavy books on your hands. They should be heavy enough to test your strength. If you have no heavy books, then try filling a large jug, vase or bowl with water. The object is to train your muscles to hold and support your partner's weight for a fairly long time. Start with five minutes and each day add five minutes to the time and another book/jug of water to the weight.

The evening exercises are more of a meditation and consist of both partners sitting opposite each other crossed-legged with a small cushion supporting the feet in position. Between you have a small bell. Make sure it has a sweet tone and is not harsh-sounding to the ears. On the man's right there is a collection of symbols. The first should be a seven-stringed vina. If you can obtain one on loan then by all means do so, if not then I suggest that you make a seven-branched symbol from florist wire and cover the wire itself with gold ribbon. If you are unable to do this, look around local shops for leaves/branches of artificial trees and make what you need from them. You can sometimes find them already in silver and gold material for special occasion bouquets. Make sure there

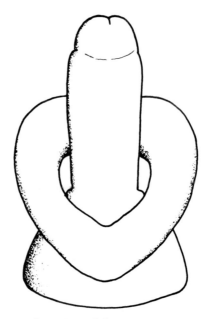

*Figure 10:* Lingam and yoni model

are *seven* branches. The second symbol is a golden lotus flower. This can be made from gold-coloured paper quite easily. The third symbol is a small sword – or a dagger will do just as well.

On the woman's left there are also three symbols: an egg which has been 'blown' and painted gold, a conch shell (there are specialist shops dealing in exotic shells and corals, but if you cannot find one then use a smaller one but make sure it has a long spiral shape) and a trident cut from strong card and covered with silver foil. If you have the skill to make one from wood or metal then do so, but it must be painted silver. These are the symbols of Brahma, Vishnu and Shiva respectively. During the week of preparation you will also need to make a lingam surrounded by the yoni out of modelling clay (see Fig 10). Paint them in one of the following colour combinations:

1) Gold and silver.
2) Blue and red.
3) White, black and red.

During the week you will have read about the three divine couples and will now be ready to meditate on each one. The woman rings the bell once, then both partners begin to assume the God forms of the first couple, Brahma and Saraswati. Start by opening the centres from the crown of the head to the genitals, then simultaneously draw light from the first and last centres opened towards the heart centre and there let them fuse together in a flame. From the intense light created by this fusion form a small figure of Brahma in the male partner's and Saraswati in the female partner's heart centre.

When the image has stabilized allow these images to grow until slightly under the size of the human form. Remember two things:

1) *You* must always be in full control.
2) These two God forms are benevolent and creative and will not harm you.

*Saraswati begins the invocation, giving to her consort the symbol of the golden egg.*

*Saraswati:* Thou art Brahma the Creator and all things are willed by thee. Out of thy substance came space, out of space came air, out of air came fire, out of fire came water and out of water, earth. From thee came the force of life. I see thee before me and the light of a thousand suns shines from thee.

*Brahma places the egg to his left side and gives to Saraswati the sacred vina/seven-branched symbol.*

*Brahma:* Thou art Saraswati, thou art the creatrix of all things and together we are one. From thee comes all knowledge and the 64 arts are the rewards of those who worship thee. Thou art the mother of the Vedas, thou art the auspicious one. Together we have created all things and the light within thee is like unto a thousand moons.

*Saraswati places the symbol to her right and they allow their respective God forms to dissolve back into the flame of the heart centre. After a short pause the women rings the bell twice. Both form the second divine couple from the heart flame, Vishnu within the man and Laxshmi within the woman. When they are fully centred Vishnu presents Laxshmi with the golden lotus.*

*Vishnu:* How beautiful thou art, fair as a garden of fragrant flowers. Thou art an instrument of exquisite pleasure whose harmonies fill the universe with beauty. Nothing can surpass thee, thou art perfection.

*Laxshmi places the lotus to her right side, takes up the conch shell and offers it to Vishnu.*

*Laxshmi:* Thou art the preserver of life. If I am the instrument of pleasure, then thine is the hand that plays the melody. No music is heard that comes not from our joining, without Vishnu and Laxshmi nothing will grow or prosper, and there will be no love and no fertility.

*There is a pause during which the God forms are allowed to dissolve into the heart flame. Then the third and last of the divine partners are built up. Kali rings the bell three times, she then picks up the trident and gives it to her Shakta, Shiva.*

Kali: Shiva, Lord of Life, Lord of the Three Worlds, Master of the Infinite Cosmos, prepare thyself for my coming, for out of thy divine body will I, Kali, create thy life anew. In union with thee at the point of death and transcendence shall I dance the great dance that knoweth no ending and all that lives shall share our joy.

*Shiva places the trident on his left side and passes the sword to Kali.*

Shiva: Divine Kali, thou of whom humanity knows so little and fears so much, thou for whom I gladly transcend life and enter the state of ecstasy, begin thy dance of love upon my body and together we shall tread the path of *shushumna.*

*The images are then allowed to return to the heart flame and the uniting flame returns to the crown and genital chakras. Close all the centres firmly and return to full consciousness.*

This is a fairly long and rather taxing evening session but it will help you to acquire the stamina for the day-long ritual to come. You will find many translations of the sacred Hindu books in which you can read the invocations and prayers to this triune male/female God form.

Lotus is a good body oil to use for this ritual, and you can match it with a lotus incense. There are also many tapes of suitable music now available which you can use to heighten the effect. The intention of this long and difficult rite is to bring about a cosmic awareness of the inextricably entwined male/female deities of the Hindu triad and the fact that their powers lie hidden in every man and woman, and indeed in all living creatures. It is a fact seldom faced by humanity that it is not the only living species on this planet that holds a minute part of the original body of the Creator, that every living thing is a chalice for that divine life force. The words 'In so much as ye have done unto them, so ye have done so unto me' hold true in the vivisection laboratory as well as in the torture chamber. There is nothing to choose between them, and those who deal in death and pain will face the black side of Kali in due time.

Follow the same procedures as before with regard to the cleansing of the sacred location, i.e. bedroom, and the need for privacy. If two or more couples intend working on these rituals then the responsibility of looking after children could perhaps be shared with one couple working the ritual and the others acting as child minders.

Place a large scented candle at each corner of the room and surround it with flowers, leaves and fruit. Cover the floor with a blanket and place over this a white sheet. Use all your cushions and/or pillows to make a soft and luxurious couch. At one side on a low table place a jug of warm water and a bowl (you may have the water in a Thermos so that it will keep warm) and some soft cloths for washing and drying. You will need a bottle of lotus oil and a bottle of almond or olive oil to act as a carrier. Lay out the paired symbols in the order to be used: the golden egg and the vina, the conch shell and the lotus, the trident and the sword.

In the times between the three distinct phases of the ritual do not dress in everyday clothes but wear a light caftan, preferably of an opaque material through which the body may be outlined. This will help to keep the state of awareness going between the divine couple. No housework and only the simplest cooking is to be done during this day so all meals should be simple, sparse and prepared beforehand as far as possible. Rice dishes mixed with vegetables and diced chicken, fruit, sweet bread rolls with humus, small savoury biscuits with various toppings, and if you like yoghurt a bowl of your favourite flavour with some sweet biscuits to dip into it. A light wine, some herb teas and bottles of mineral water will complete your dietary needs.

The day will start very early, beginning at sunrise, and not end until sunset, so prepare as much as you can the evening before. Try to rise about one hour before dawn. Strip your bed of the covers used during the night and cover it with just one sheet. On the bed place the model you have made of the joined lingam and yoni and place a yellow flower before it. Spend a few moments in silent meditation before this symbol. Bathe and wash your hair, eat some fruit and drink some water or herb tea, then go and stand together before a window and watch the moment of dawn approach. The ritual begins from this moment.

# The Dance of Love

## Place on the Tree = Hod. Keynote = Transcendence Through Mental Power.

*The couple hold hands facing each other and after a few moments walk to the prepared couch. The man sits down, leaning back against the cushions, feet and legs apart displaying the sacred lingam. The woman stands before him feet slightly apart with her fingers interlaced in the Mudra of the Mahayoni, the gesture of the Great Mother Goddess Saraswati/Laxshmi/ Kali (see Fig 11). Slowly she rises on the balls of the feet and bends her knees, keeping the back straight, until she is in a squatting position. She speaks.*

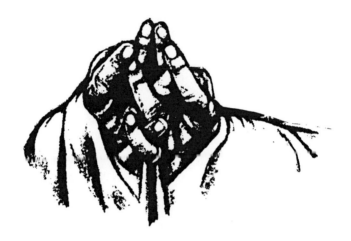

*Figure 11:* The gesture of the Great Mother Goddess

*Saraswati:* Brahma, awake from thy dream at the request of the mother. It is time for a new universe to be created. Awake and by the power of the sacred lingam and yoni all things shall be renewed and made whole.

*She returns to the standing position and Brahma awakes and stands with her. He caresses her slowly over her whole body, saying:*

*Brahma:* Saraswati, Shakti of Brahma, radiant being of my soul, thou art together with me and we are one being.

*They hold each other closely as if one person.*

*Both:* To make a new universe there must be a division between us, male and female must we be to create life.

*They separate slowly, Brahma to sit as before displaying the lingam. Saraswati takes up the oil and pours a little into her hand. She kneels before Brahma and takes the lingam between her hands, smoothing the oil into it and into the testicles, encouraging Brahma to erection.*

*Saraswati:* Only I, Saraswati, may call forth the creative power of Brahma. Only I may dance the dance of bringing into being with him. I am Saraswati, the mother of the Vedas, the auspicious one, the teacher of the 64 arts. Awake to my caresses, O Brahma, and let the dance begin.

*She ceases her caresses and kisses the head of the lingam in adoration, then in her turn lies back against the cushions to await the attention of Brahma. He pours some oil into his hands and kneels before his consort Shakti Saraswati. He in turn begins to oil and caress the yoni, bringing the Goddess to a state of sexual readiness.*

*Brahma:* Thou art the seven ecstasies of union, thou art the holder of life, the singer of sweet songs. In union with thee my body becomes a temple of joy. Wrapped in the arms of Saraswati, Brahma knows only the infinite ecstasy of creation.

*He kisses the sacred yoni of the Goddess in adoration and they both rise to a sitting lotus position. Using the techniques of assumption practised during the evening exercises, they open the centres from the crown of the head to the genitals and bring the two golden rays of light together in the heart flame. From this they build the God/Goddess images within and allow them to assume nearly full size. The man contemplates his partner as Saraswati the golden Goddess, and she sees him as Brahma the golden God. Brahma takes up the golden egg and presents it to Saraswati. She gives him the vina. The couple must hold on to the indwelling God forms as strongly as possible. When ready they lay aside the sacred symbols and Saraswati lies back on her cushions raising her legs to set her feet on Brahma's shoulders. The God moves forward, lifting her hips so that they rest upon his lower thighs. Using his fingers he opens the yoni of Saraswati with a gentle touch, remembering how delicate the inner labia can be. His control both of the inner image and the power of the lingam must be absolute at this moment. The head of the lingam enters. Brahma pauses and speaks:*

*Brahma:* I have made the starry void and separated the earth from the waters. Great is the power of Brahma and Saraswati.

*Saraswati:* I have formed the mountains and the seas, the valleys and the lakes. Together we are all powerful.

*The lingam enters further and Brahma pauses and says:*

*Brahma:* I have created the sun and the clouds, the thunder and the lightning, and all the precious things found in the earth.

*Saraswati:* I have formed the moon from the pearls of the oceans and the growing things of earth. Rejoice with me, my love.

*The lingam enters further still and Brahma pauses to say:*

*Brahma:* All creatures that fly and swim and walk upon the earth have I made. They shall make their own kind and shall cover the earth with life in many forms.

*Saraswati:* The earth lies waiting for the coming of the children of Brahma and Saraswati. Sow the seed that shall form them.

*Brahma enters the Goddess fully and she crosses her ankles behind his neck and extends her arms to the sides and grasps the symbols of the divine couple. Now the Gods enter completely into union and the inner images must be held as clearly as possible with no thought of self. As the final moment draws near the two must use all their control to pause at the last moment and visualize their bodies as interwoven energy patterns rather than bodies, then as the sexual climax is allowed to flower both must flow with the released energy like a golden river down into the earth. Offer all that is flowing to the divine couple for them to use as they will. It is important to try to 'keep flying' as long as possible. Brahma now*

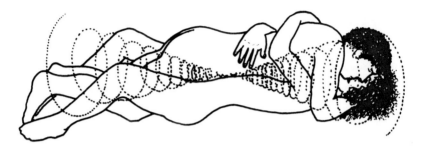

*Figure 12:* Spiral energy

*sinks down upon the breast of Saraswati and they rest. At this time they are free to absorb the residue of the divine energies they have offered to the Gods. This is done by aligning their navels so they touch and allowing the last of the energy to mingle and travel through their bodies in a spiral form (see Fig 12). Then the inner images may return to the heart flame and wait there.*

*When fully rested they bathe each other with warm scented water, drink wine or tea, and eat if they wish. Then together they sit in silent worship of the lingam/yoni symbol until the desire to rebuild the images of Brahma and Saraswati awakens. Together they recall the God forms and contemplate the divine in themselves. Place the full attention on specific parts of the partner's body and try to recall its inner energy pattern. Music is helpful at this time and a quiet reading of the Vedas, or a reading from the* Kama Sutra.

*The woman may feel a desire to dance at this stage and should obey this inner urging. Dance is a way of expressing joy, vitality and love. Use your whole body to say exactly what you are feeling at the moment or to convey a message to your partner. Remember that the dancer is a powerful archetype.*

*Pass the time quietly until the approach of noon, then about half an hour before move into the lotus position facing each other and allow the Brahma and Saraswati images to return to the heart flame. Refill the linked centres with new energy and see the heart flames flare up again, only this time they are blue.*

*Within the flames build up the images of Vishnu and Laxshmi within and take on the God forms of 'the Eternal Lovers', as they are called. When the assumption is complete, the second part of the ritual may start. It is said that Vishnu the Lover has so much energy that he can make love to a hundred women . . . he can, but they are all Laxshmi for she is all women. She is above all the initiatress of sexual love.*

*The ritual begins with the enticement of Vishnu by his Shakti. She uses all her powers: dance, music, love play, words, caresses and mock refusal.*

*This should go on until the beloved can stand no more teasing and catches her and brings her to the couch. They stand close together and she brings one leg up and around his hip/thigh. Both her hands rest lightly on his shoulders and Vishnu fills her vagina with his erect phallus.*

*In this position the love play begins.*

*Vishnu:* Thou art like a tall lotus flower growing up to the sun, but I shall cut thee down with a sharp thrust.

*Laxshmi:* I shall grow again, O best beloved, and take another form for thee. Against my woman's power Vishnu must fall.

*She retreats from his phallus and draws him down to the floor. If her hair is long she throws it over her head and draws it down his body, winding it around his erection and slowly allowing it to unwind as she pulls away. If it is not long enough then she uses her hands, fingers and lips to achieve the same result. Kneeling over him, she inserts the phallus into her vagina and slowly descends upon him, using circular and undulating movements of her hips and thighs to perform the dance of Laxshmi.*

*Laxshmi:* Vishnu, preserver of life, let me know thy power, let me adore thee and fill thee with the energies of the Shakti Laxshmi. Thou art made from the blue flame of self creation as I am made of the red flame of love. Together we shall create an undying fire.

*Vishnu:* Lady of beauty, let me know thy sweetness, let me touch the inner petals of thy sacred chakra with the lingam and fill the vase of life to overflowing. Thy hands are cool with scented oil and thy lips are warm with wine.

*The Goddess withdraws the phallus from her body and goes to fetch wine to share with her consort. When this has been drunk she kneels with her back to him and offers herself, looking back over her shoulder and smiling. Vishnu kneels on one knee behind her, the other close to her hip, one arm goes over her right shoulder, the hand cupping her left breast, the left arm goes around her left hip, the hand pressing firmly between her thighs. In this position he enters the Goddess.*

*Vishnu:* Thus I will claim thee for my beloved. Thy heart is mine, thy flower is mine, thy yoni is mine and this moment shall be preserved in time.

*Laxshmi:* I am part of thee as thou are part of me also. I cannot be claimed, only made whole as once we were before creation began. We are one being, for am I not also Saraswati and Kali, are you not also Brahma and Shiva, and if I am also you and you are me, then we are truly one and indivisible.

*The Goddess withdraws from Vishnu and turns to help him lie down with his knees drawn up slightly. She mounts, facing him, her knees on either side of his hips and leans back a little against his knees. Her arms, holding the golden lotus and the conch shell, are extended above her head and in this position they move towards the climax of their union. Laxshmi should make good use of her inner muscles to grip the phallus as strongly as she can. With practice she should be able to hold it in her so tightly her partner cannot withdraw. But remember the phallus is delicate and can be easily bruised. (The pathworking can be used during this part of the ritual if it is so wished.)*

Vishnu: I see the sun approach and fill me with fire. The golden lotus opens its petals to me, I become its stem and its root. I am the earth beneath the flower, from me it rises up and blooms in beauty fed by the waters of my seed.

Laxshmi: I hear the inner music of the sea. The shell speaks to me and in its secret cavity I hear the rushing of the inner waters. I am the lotus, I am the lotus, I am the lotus, and within me lies the secret of life.

*Both partners should hold to their inner images of the God forms as the climax sweeps through them. As they rest, they may absorb the power left over after the Gods have accepted their offering. Using warm water they then bathe each other and drink some water and eat some fruit. It would be advisable to sleep a little now, but if not, then rest quietly on the bed until you feel like eating the second meal of the day.*

*This last part of the day leading up to sunset and the final part of the ritual is likely to be the hardest. The God forms must be kept as close to the surface of consciousness as possible. Thoughts, actions, words and pastimes should be part of the role-playing. Reading can be used, also listening to music and quiet meditation. No one said it would be easy, but until you have attempted this ritual you will not fully understand how hard it can be to keep a God form uppermost in the conscious mind.*

*Make sure the sacred place is tidy: clean up any unwanted debris, shake up the pillows and cushions, take away empty glasses, cups and plates. Refill clean glasses with wine and fill the water jug. Change the sheet covering the 'couch' for a clean one and sprinkle fresh herbs and/or flower petals over it. Westerners can find it very hard to relax and do nothing but concentrate on sexual build up and the retention of God forms for a whole day. They may find it hard not to switch on the television to see how their favourite football team is doing or may feel a need to phone a friend, start baking, or even weeding the garden. Resist these urges or you will undo all the good you have achieved so far.*

*The last part of the ritual will be the hardest, and the God forms the most difficult to build and hold. About half an hour before sunset sit facing each other and allow the God forms of Vishnu and Laxshmi to return into the blue heart flame. Meditate for a few minutes on Shiva as the Lord of Transcendence and Kali as the Liberator of Souls. Then allow the two rays of light to rush towards each other from the head chakra and the genital chakra and unite in a brilliant red and white flame. Out of this flame emerge the Gods, building up until they almost fill the bodies of their respective worshippers.*

*Wait for a moment to allow the distinctive passions of Shiva and Kali to arise. Shiva's power is that of ecstasy, a feeling that cannot be fully* described, only felt, only experienced. His is the ultimate sacrifice of life for love, yet in the dying he lives from age to age.

Kali is pure passion, insatiable and destructive, yet she also has a softer image, Parvati the ultimate woman. These two images will alternate through this part of the ritual and must be controlled at all times. These are the two God forms that will bring this ritual to its conclusion.

Shiva rises and begins to stamp and dance.

Shiva: I am Shiva, lord of life, the dreamer of dreams, the supreme yogi, lord of all creatures, the ageless dancer. I am the deathless one. I am the lord of Meru, master of austerity.

He stops and looks down at Kali and speaks to her. She kneels at his feet and places her hands upon them.

Shiva: Thou art my precious one, my jewel, the incomparable lady of joy. Without you I would have no power in the world of men. Into thy hands I place my body. Let it be thy toy Kali, lady of perfume and sweet odours.

He sits down, feet lightly crossed at the ankles, leaning back on his arms. The sacred lingam is exposed to Kali's gaze. She kneels to worship the lingam and then raises herself above Shiva. With her feet on either side of his thighs, she lowers herself slowly onto the waiting lingam, then raises her arms, opens her eyes wide, and thrusts out her tongue. Shiva sits up and clasps her about the waist, supporting her weight. Her legs now slide around him and she is thus seated astride him in sexual union. Shiva leans forward and touches her tongue with his. They remain motionless with the upright phallus completely penetrating the vagina. Kali holds Shiva's head against her shoulder or breast. Using only her inner muscles, Kali begins the dance of ecstasy whilst Shiva remains absolutely still. She must pause the moment she feels the slightest movement of the phallus or if she starts to climax and wait until the moment dies away.

Kali: I am the scabbard to thy sword, O Shiva. I am thy protection against all who would disturb thee. I am the flame of love and the taker of strength. I am the giver of blessings and the destroyer of life. I shall take thy life, Shiva.

She rises from Shiva and begins to dance around him in a circle. Taking up her sword, she mimes the cutting off of Shiva's head. Her attitude must be threatening and full of female power. Every now and then she takes on one of Kali's postures (see Fig 9). Finally she lays Shiva out as if he were indeed dead and stands over him exulting.

Kali: I am thy death, I am the cause and the triumph of thy transcendence. I am thy love, thy destroyer, thy path of shu-shumna. I am Kali, I am that without which nothing can enter the realms of the eternal. I claim thy life, Shiva, I will empty thee of thy force.

She sits over the recumbent God and sheathes his erect phallus in her vagina. Shiva must allow Kali to be the only one to move for as long as he can. *The longer he can refrain from thrusting the more powerful will be the climax. Kali's purpose is to call forth the seed of Shiva in order that he may live again through his own life force. Kali must continue to move and to chant the names of the three Gods, Brahma, Vishnu, Shiva, until the moment of climax, when she must draw up the seed into her body and hold her muscles tight keeping the emission locked into her body, then relax and allow the fluid to drain downwards covering the body of Shiva.*

*Kali:* Shiva, my love and my lord, rise up and live. I pour out the force of life upon thee. I summon thee from the shadows by the sacred *mudras.*

*She places the palms of her hands around the phallus of Shiva. This is the* yoni *mudra. Then, holding the phallus in her right hand and extending the left beneath the tooticles, which is the* lingam *mudra, finally she forms the* mahayoni *mudra with interlaced fingers (see Fig 11).*

*Shiva wakes, rises to his feet and places his right hand between the breasts of Kali.*

*Shiva:* Hail, thou giver of life, dancer of the void, Goddess of power, Kali Yurga.

*She offers him wine and bathes him as he drinks, then bathes herself. They then sit facing and allow the God forms to return to the heart flames and close down all the centres firmly. Food, some tea and sleep is recommended after this; however it sometimes happens that the woman will be restless during the night after such a ritual. If so, do not try to sleep, but get up and drain the excess energy in dance or vigorous exercise, then return to bed.*

# The Pathworking

(This pathworking can be done sitting in the usual God form position and separately, or it can be made a part of the morning or afternoon ongoing work of the ritual itself. In the latter case it will increase its power if used *during* the Vishnu/Laxshmi union as indicated.)

Visualize a cloud of blue mist descending towards the earth. It comes to rest on a pathway beaten into the soil by the passing of many feet. On the right side the earth slopes down towards a wide slow-moving river, and on the left there are fields that give way to a large tropical forest.

From the blue mist there comes the sound of a flute. For several moments we listen to it playing and enjoying the subtle harmonies invented by the hidden musician. Then from the mist there steps a man, tall and dark-haired, supple of body, graceful in his movements and with an air of greatness about him. His skin is blue and he wears embroidered trousers and a loose-fitting coat of thin white wool. He begins to walk along the path, still playing the flute.

From the trees the birds answer the silver notes and animals look up from their feeding as he goes by. Suddenly he stops playing and looks towards the forest. Coming across the fields is a beautiful girl. Her skin is soft and her eyes large and clear, her breasts are full and firm and her waist narrow, her hips are curved and move with enticing grace beneath her pleated skirt. She is singing as she walks towards us.

Vishnu, for he is the flute player, begins to play again, this time imitating the girl's voice with little grace notes. She sees him and stops to listen and then comes towards him laughing. He calls her by name for it is his beloved consort and Shakti who stands before him. Together they walk along the path until they come to a place of green grass and brilliant flowers. There Vishnu sits down and draws Laxshmi to his right and begins to caress her. Laxshmi sings of her love for Vishnu and together they call the other Gods to witness their eternal devotion to each other. In the distance they hear the sound of little bells and down the road come 50 beautiful women. Each one is different but all are exquisite in their loveliness. There are silver bells tied to their feet and wrists and their eyes are darkened with kohl and their hands and feet patterned with henna. Reaching the divine couple they surround them, singing and dancing in a circle.

These are the Gopis, the milk-maids who wait upon Vishnu when he appears upon the earth. Laxshmi stands up and begins to dance. Round and round she goes, telling with her hands, eyes and movements ancient stories of love and passion. Now we begin to see that we were wrong in thinking each of the dancing Gopis were different, now we see that they are all the same, all Laxshmi in her many manifestations. She is wife, lover, whore, mother, virgin, girl child, old woman; she is black, and white and golden. As they circle around him Vishnu sees them as the stars, each one dancing the appointed pattern and forming future possibilities by their grouping. In the middle is the lovely Laxshmi, the centre of and a part of them all.

Now she approaches her consort and begins to disrobe before him. He lays aside the flute and waits for her to come to him, knowing her to be his inner self, as he is her other self. As she takes him into her the Gopis disappear, becoming one with the Goddess. In silent union the Eternal Lovers begin the sacred breath. A change comes over them and they begin to transform into Shiva and Parvati. The scenery changes also and becomes a tall mountain, cloud-peaked and snow-capped, the sacred Mount Meru where the Gods of change and death have their abode.

Shiva stands up, lifting Parvati with him. Her head is thrown back and her arms are about his neck. The union continues and deepens and the chant of many voices can be heard upon the winds that blow about the summit of the sacred mountain. Shiva's body begins to glow and becomes radiant. He begins to transcend the physical body. Slowly he lifts Parvati from him and sets her down, then he falls to the ground and the radiance that is all about him consumes all that is of the earth and he is left apparently lifeless. Parvati also changes and her body becomes black and four-armed. Her face is fierce and her tongue lashes out like that of a lion scenting its prey. Around her waist is a circle of skulls and in one hand she holds a sword and in another a lifeless head that drips blood. She has become Kali the Slayer.

She begins to dance the Great Dance of Life and Death. We see that despite the sword and the head her other two hands are held out in blessing and protection. 'Fear me not,' she seems to say to us, 'for I am that which is eternal and I come to show you that all is well and in death shall all humanity become like Gods.'

Her dance takes her to the body of her Shakta and she stands upon him and lowers herself until the lingam and the yoni are conjoined. A flash of light blinds us for a moment and, when we can see again, before us stand Brahma the Creator and the gentle Saraswati. They shine with a golden light and smile upon those before them. They hold out their arms and draw us towards them. To Brahma's arms go the women and Saraswati enfolds the men. Within their divine embrace we are reborn into light and knowledge of the ultimate divinity of love and grace. We become one with them and with Shiva and Kali, Vishnu and Laxshmi and for a fleeting moment of earth's time we travel the path of *shushumna* and become one with eternity itself. In this feeling we bask and receive what is due to us as human beings that are both good and bad. Then the light dims and we feel the divine ones part from us, yet they leave behind a grain of light to keep within, to fan into a flame when we join together in the Dance of Love.

# Ritual 4

# THE RITUAL OF THE HAWTHORN TOWER

## The Programme

This ritual corresponds to the sphere of Netzach on the Tree of Life, and I have chosen to use the archetypes of Merlin and Nimuë as the *alter egos* of the participating couple. This sphere is concerned with Venus and therefore with love and with the many forms both physical and abstract that love may take. The main symbols of Netzach are the rose and the lamp, and both these appear in the ritual itself. It seemed to me to be the ideal placing for Nimuë the Enchantress who spirited Merlin away to her Hawthorn Tower in the depths of the forest, where he then became the male equivalent of Sleeping Beauty. This fairy tale echoes the myth of Diana, the Moon Goddess who fell in love with a mortal man named Endymion. Because she had sworn herself to chastity, she cast him into a deep sleep and hid him in a cave where she could visit him nightly and gaze upon him to her heart's content without breaking her vow.

The Qabalah makes Netzach the sphere of the Elohim, or the Gods, and certainly the ancient pantheons saw nothing amiss in using the gift of sexual love to the full. Both mortals and immortals indulged themselves, and according to the myths and legends the bloodlines of humans and Gods were thoroughly mixed. This sphere is also concerned with the multiplicity of forms that come from sexual pairing and this includes those who are only partly human by virtue of having one parent of fairy or non-human blood. It also includes, for the purpose of this ritual, the forms taken on by shape-changers, and both Nimuë and Merlin qualify in this respect.

In his later years Merlin was supposedly enticed by Nimuë's fairy wiles, but that makes a nonsense of his supposed wisdom and powers of observation. He is also usually presented as a grey-bearded man of great age, but there are legends that speak of him

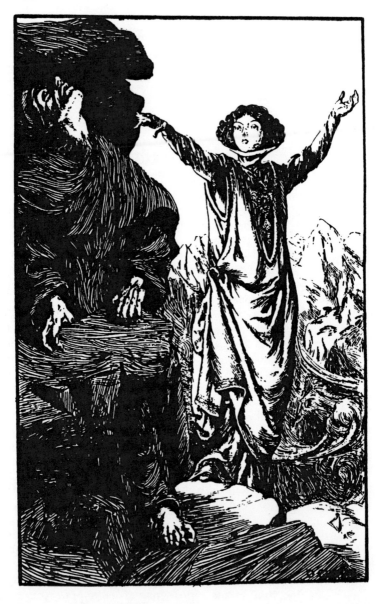

*Figure 13:* Merlin and Nimuë *(Dora Curtis,* from *An Arthurian Reader)*

as a young and handsome man, one who could and did appear in whatever guise suited his purpose. He was only part human, being the son of a human virgin and a non-human father. One story says his father was a lord of the fairy folk, another says he was sired by a demon bent on creating the Anti-Christ. This last was prevented by the hermit Blaise christening the child at birth and claiming him for the Church.

Many of the legends hint that he is celibate, while others tell of him having both a wife and a sister, and his encounter with Nimuë is very obviously a sexual one. Merlin as the archetypal magician is far older than the Arthurian cycle. His origins are lost in the mists that surround the drowned lands of Atlantis and Lyonesse. No one knows where Merlin obtained his magical training but it would be reasonable to assume that he was taught by either his non-human father or his fairy kin – or perhaps by those who had ruled the lost lands. He can also be seen as part of the monomyth of the hero or seeker, for if we look at the quest pattern we see that every seeker who achieves the quest and their heart's desire is obliged to return to the world and train a successor before they can find the way back, this time forever. I find it entirely believable that Merlin would have returned to train the young Arthur for kingship then, having succeeded in the object of his return, looked to the fairy woman Nimuë to provide him with a doorway back to Tir-nan-Og.

The intention of this ritual is for Merlin to summon the enchantress and persuade her to use her powers to open the ancient door between the worlds. It is she who holds the key that will release him from the world of men, but he must win it from her. In human terms the intention is for the woman to open the door of intuition to man.

If you intend doing this ritual outdoors then make it a weekend away and look for a place where you can find space and privacy on mountains or moorlands. Woodlands and small valleys are equally viable.

By now you know that the week before the ritual must be one of celibacy, much as you hate the thought! The preliminary exercises are quite different this time, as a complete change of direction can often prevent a slackness of concentration before it fully manifests.

Those for the woman are as follows: set your alarm for an hour before dawn every morning and get up at once – if you stop to think about it you will never do it. If you have a garden or even a small yard, slip outside and stand naked, letting the cool air clothe you with the promise of morning. If you do have a garden with grass, lie down and roll in the cold moistness and let it bathe you. Cup the dew in your hands and lave your face with it. If you only have access to a yard or a balcony, then simply hold up your arms and let your spirit welcome the coming sun. If you have to be content with working indoors, stand a large jug of water on a window-ledge where the sun and the light can fill it. Then in the morning stand before an open window and let your mind's eye show you the sun coming up over mountains that glisten with snow caps. Then dip your fingers into the water and let the drops run down over your body. Do this until most of the water has been used. Towel yourself dry and sit quietly for just 10 minutes, building up an inner location of trees and rocks and winding paths that lead down into secret hollows where birds nest and small animals live. Build up the image of Nimuë as you think she is, then absorb that image and let it stay within you. Go back to bed and fix your mind on the enchantress archetype until you sleep again, willing yourself to dream of her.

The exercises for the man also require an early start. Get up with your partner but instead of bathing in the dew or washing with sun-filled water you are going to walk. If you are near a park then walk in it, slowly savouring the early morning noises and scents before the traffic fumes begin to fill the air. As you walk, imagine yourself as Merlin setting out from Camelot, knowing that you will never see it again. You are going to find Nimuë, for you have fulfilled your task, Arthur is king and you can safely turn your heart towards that place where long ago you learned your magical arts. In your mind's eye as you walk see the towers of the castle recede and the forest and mountains draw nearer. Stop now and then and listen with the inner ear for the sound of Nimuë's voice singing.

If you wish use the lovely music and lyrics given to Nimuë to sing in the musical *Camelot*. Make her voice crystal clear and silver sweet. Then make your way home again and slip back into the warm bed for a further hour to dream of a fairy woman who wears roses in her hair.

The evening exercises are also different from those previous. You will need a piece of net or veiling large enough to cover the woman to her ankles when thrown over her head, and a coronet of roses, which do not have to be real. The colour of the net should be pale green if possible, if not, then white will do. The man wears a hooded robe if he has one and the woman wears the coronet with the veiling thrown over her, beneath which she must be naked.

The curtains are open but the room unlit. Merlin sits in medita-tion recalling his time in Tir-nan-Og and those who taught him the magical arts. He should build pictures in his mind of faces and give them names as far as he is able. One face keeps returning, that of his love Nimuë as he last saw her, veiled in green silk and wearing a coronet of roses. He feels the weight of the years spent in this world and longs for the Land of the Ever Young and his former youth.

*Nimuë enters quietly and stands where Merlin can see her but too far for him to touch her. He speaks softly to her:*
Nimuë, my time here comes to an end, I long for the peace of Tir-nan-Og and for you. Open the doorway and call me to you once again.
*She does not speak. He tries again.*
Nimuë, fairy maid, love of my heart, have you forgotten me, has the time been so long since we last met that my face no longer appears in your dreams?
*She does not speak, he tries a third time.*
If I must live out my life here in the world of men, without your love and your presence, then I pray you leave me a token of remembrance that will recall our love.
*She brings from beneath her veil a red rose and lets it fall to the ground. Then she withdraws and leaves Merlin to sit with the rose in his hand remembering the past.*

All this should be built with intention and both must work on the assumption that they *are* Merlin and Nimuë. Each night the same pathworking is enacted and a new rose given. These must be collected and kept fresh in water. On the last night Nimuë comes close to Merlin, lifts the veil away from her and says to the third question:

Merlin, tomorrow you must seek the gate to the Hawthorn Tower. Beyond that lies the door to Tir-nan-Og, but once you enter the tower you will be lost to the world. Think on this and be prepared to either leave this level of existence forever and be with me, or remain and pass into the unknown when your time is over.

Then she withdraws.
The ritual may be worked either in the late afternoon near sunset or in the early evening, but on a growing moon. If you are outdoors you will need wood-cloaks, a lantern, the roses and some extra rose petals, a staff for Merlin, something to lie on, and some hawthorn branches or branches of anything that has thorns or rough twigs, enough of them to build a barrier through which you will have to push your way. If the outdoor site is a good one, there will be bushes that will act as the hawthorn barrier. Make certain there is a space large enough to work in comfortably, and collect small branches and leaves to make a bed. Cover it with the folded blanket, sprinkling the extra rose petals over it. Nimuë

stands well beyond the hawthorn doorway and if possible hidden from sight. Merlin will approach carrying the lantern and the roses, which should be real.

If you are working indoors you can use the bedroom (the room must be cleared as for the other rituals) and only Merlin will need a cloak, as Nimuë can wear just the veil. The branches can be placed so that they bar the way to the room with Merlin on the other side. The extra rose petals are to be sprinkled over the bed.

The outdoor version of the rite needs nothing in the way of oils or incenses, but if worked inside they can be used with great effect. I would suggest the Sacred Wood incense, which is simply scrapings of rowan, apple, juniper, cedar, pine, holly, willow, oak and hawthorn. Others that can be used are cherry, dogwood, elder and hazel.[1]

If you intend to use music as an atmospheric aid, then look around for something with a slightly medieval sound to it. There are many tapes of this kind now available. The symbols to use for this ritual are the red rose, the lamp, the hawthorn staff and the standing stone.

# The Ritual of the Hawthorn Tower

## Sphere = Netzach. Keynote = Life and Love In All Their Forms.

*The procedure for the outdoor ritual is as follows: Nimuë goes first and takes up her station out of sight and well beyond the barrier of hawthorn. Behind her will be the 'bower' made of branches and leaves, etc. If possible this should be built against a background covering of bushes so that it provides some sort of covering, a Hawthorn Tower in fact. If you wish, a bottle of wine can be made part of the ritual, in which case you will need a cup or chalice.*

*Merlin should be some five or six minutes' walk away. In a bag or pouch slung over his shoulder he carries the roses given to him by Nimuë. He wears a robe but with nothing beneath it, sandals and his wood-cloak. He has a staff in one hand and leans heavily on it, for he is now old and tired. In the other hand he carries a lamp or lantern. He must spend a few minutes assuming the form of Merlin who, having completed his work as tutor to the Once and Future King, now seeks his own reward, the door to Tir-nan-Og. As he walks he looks around constantly as if trying to*

---

[1] For more information about Sacred Wood incenses, their meanings and use write to Dusty Miller at the address given on page 68, note 1.

*remember landmarks of long ago. He will make three stops before finally coming to the Hawthorn Tower. The first stop.*

*Merlin:* Things are so changed I scarce remember the path that once I trod with the vigour of youth. Nimuë, Nimuë, hear me, fairy maid, and guide my footsteps to the door I seek.

*He listens for a while.*

There is no answer to my call.

*He walks on a while and then stops again.*

Nimuë, Nimuë, my lost love, hear me, I beg you. Do not forget your promise to open the door to youth and joy once my task was completed. Arthur rules as high king and needs me no more.

*He listens again but there is only silence. He walks on until he is near to the hawthorn barrier and then stops for the third time and calls out:*

Aengus Og, Lord of the Sidhe, father, once I sat at your table and learned from the wise men of ancient Atlantis who had sought refuge with you. Hear me now, send Nimuë to me that she may open the emerald door to the Land of the Heart's Desire. I, Merlin, son of Aengus Og and the last priestess of Atlantis, call for aid in my quest.

*Nimuë calls from beyond the barrier:*

*Nimuë:* Who calls me with a voice so like the one I knew long years past? Who walks the paths of the Lady of the Woods?

*Merlin comes closer and calls out:*

*Merlin:* Nimuë, it is I, Merlin, come to redeem my promise that I would come again and woo you for my own once my great task was done. Open the Hawthorn Tower, sweet Nimuë, and let me pass through into your arms.

*Nimuë:* Merlin was my love, lost to me in the world of men. He set forth upon a quest to aid the High King of Albion but no word has come from him and I fear that death, both the boon and the bane of men, has taken him.

*Merlin:* Not so Nimuë, I am Merlin come again to claim thee for my love.

*Nimuë comes to the hawthorn barrier and sees him.*

*Nimuë:* This is not my love, the strong and handsome youth who won my heart. You are heavy with mortal years and close to that which men call death. I will not open the doorway for such as you.

*Merlin:* Nimuë, I swear by the hooded falcon I gave thee at our first trysting, 'Speedwing' you named it, that I am that same Merlin.

*Nimuë:* That name you had from some knight at Arthur's court who knew my love. I believe you not.

*Merlin:* I swear that I am Merlin by the green garter that I bound about your knee on a May morning long ago, knotting in its ribbons a lock of my hair and of yours.

*Nimuë:* Ah, cruel tongue that gossips of our ways of love to others, how else can you know of this? Go hence, stay not on fairy ground.

*Merlin:* Sweet guardian of my heart, I swear that I am that same Merlin that caught thy virgin blood upon the petals of a white rose and by magical art set it in a crystal to last forever. That same crystal you keep beneath your pillow at night. Now I come to reclaim what it holds.

*Nimuë comes close to the barrier.*

*Nimuë:* It *is* you, my dear love, but how changed by the world of men. I did dream for a full seven days that you called me, but thought it just a fancy of my heart. Come, I will open up the gate of thorn, but first you must give up that weary shell and leave it behind.

*Merlin:* I will bring with me only the roses you gave to me in dream, made real by my art, and this lamp I will leave here upon this tree. It will point the way to fairyland for all true lovers who pass this way.

*He sheds the wood-cloak and, carrying the roses, approaches the hawthorn barrier.*

*Merlin:* By the power of the first rose I shed my human years and restore my youth. By the power of the second rose I leave the world of men behind. By the power of the third rose I bind my heart to thine. By the power of the fourth rose I will become my father's liegeman. By the power of the fifth rose I pledge to teach from the inner levels any who will seek me as a teacher and who will take on the quest. By the power of the sixth rose I vow to go to the aid of Albion should the need arise in the future. By the power of the seventh rose I will take thee, Nimuë, to wife until this eternity be done and beyond. Open the door to me, beloved.

*Nimuë comes and pulls aside the barrier. Merlin pushes through, daring the few thorns that still bar his way, and stands before her. He lifts her veil and lets it fall to the ground so that she is dressed in just the coronet of roses and her own beauty. He kneels before her.*

*Merlin:* My lady and my love, to thee I offer my heart and service. Never again shall we be parted, for my quest ends here and I have returned.

*Nimuë takes the lamp, leads Merlin to the bower and hangs the lamp nearby.*

*Nimuë:* Merlin, the lamp and the rose are the symbols of love and in the presence of those symbols I shall take you for my lord and my companion. In their presence will you take me for your lady and your love?

*Merlin:* This is my desire and my intention and by the rose and the lamp I pledge myself to thee.

*Nimuë lies down on the prepared bed and Merlin takes the seven roses and lays the head of one between her breasts, another on her belly and a third between her thighs. The rest he scatters as petals all over her body. He kneels at her feet, lifts each foot in turn to his lips and kisses the sole, then each knee, the rose of the clitoris set within its own hawthorn barrier, the belly, each breast and finally her lips.*

*Merlin:* Thus do I worship thee and bless each part of thee. I name thee my rose of love, my lamp of blessedness.

*Nimuë now rises, lays Merlin down upon the bed and kneels at his feet. She follows the same pattern, kissing the soles of his feet, his knees, scrotum, phallus, belly, breast and lips.*

*Nimuë:* I bless your body with my body, I worship your passion with my passion. You are the sword and I am its scabbard. You are the dagger and I the chalice. Give to me and I shall receive and return in another form.

*She sinks down upon him, taking him into her body until fully sheathed, then she stretches her arms upwards and calls upon the stars to witness their love.*

Behold me, ye watchers of the night, I am Nimuë and Merlin is my love.

*The mating begins and the pair must keep the* alter egos *of Nimuë and Merlin as fully as possible. Do not hurry, but allow the pleasure to rise slowly, and while it is still possible, pause and hold the moment. Nimuë leans back on her arms and lets her head drop back, her hair sweeping Merlin's thighs.*

*Nimuë:* Let Tir-nan-Og rejoice in the mating of Nimuë and Merlin.

*For the second time the mating proceeds and the moment allowed to rise, then another pause.*

*Nimuë:* To the power of Aengus Og, Lord of the Sidhe, is the gift of this mating given.

*The mating proceeds to the end, the power is offered and accepted. The pair should then rest and wrap themselves warmly against a chill. Wine may be shared at this point. If there is the desire, a second mating for the couple alone will make a perfect ending to the ritual. The rose heads should be dipped in the mingled body fluids and buried at the site, and if possible some flower seeds scattered over them. Then dress and clear the site and return home. If worked indoors simply adapt the outdoor instructions to suit your environment.*

# The Pathworking

You stand in a moonlit garden filled with the scent of flowers. Above you a new moon floats serenely in the midnight sky and the gentle sounds of night-time can be heard. You are Merlin, the son of Aengus Og and this is Tir-nan-Og, the Land of the Ever Young, where you have been tutored on the arts of magic for the last five years. Your destiny has been set out for you from the moment of conception. On your shoulders lies the responsibility for the training of the High King of Britain, Arthur, the Once and Future King. For many years you have studied and prepared and learned from the wise men who once taught in the drowned lands of the West. Your human mother came from those lands long ago as a priestess from the Temple of Naradek and chose to join her ancient bloodline to that of Aengus Og, Lord of the Sidhe, in order to bring you to birth.

You look up at the great castle walls, see the pennant flying from the topmost tower and sigh. Soon you will be leaving this land of fairy and taking up your appointed task. Inside the castle a great feast is being held for you, a farewell before you leave to live among ordinary men and women, but you are here to take a more private farewell.

From a small door in the castle comes a young girl, a maiden of the Sidhe, tall and slender with hair the colour of a blackbird's wing and eyes as green as the depths of the sea. She comes hurrying through the garden looking from side to side, searching for her love who is soon to leave her for long weary years, the span of a human lifetime. Nimuë sees you and runs into your arms holding you close. Her cloudy hair lies loose upon her shoulders, bound by a coronet of deep creamy white roses, and their scent fills the air about you. You know you will always carry this picture of her in your heart. You draw her deeper into the gardens towards a small arbour where moonflowers bloom and scent the night.

There is so much to say and so little time in which to say it: lovers down through the ages have never had enough time. You tell Nimuë of your love for her and ask her to wait until your time in the world has come to an end. Your father has promised that once the appointed task has been completed you may return to Tir-nan-Og, and when that time comes you will not leave again and you will ask her to be your wife. In the Undying Lands she will still be as young as she is now, and you, although old in human terms, will be made young again by the magic of the land itself.

Tonight belongs to the two of you, it is all you will have to remember when you leave, a memory that will have to last a human lifetime until the day you meet again. Within the arbour all is quiet and the feasting and the music seem far away, there is just you and Nimuë, your dear love.

Her kisses are sweeter than the finest fairy wine and you feel you could exist on these alone, not caring for food. But kisses are not enough and the night becomes a shield for love as Nimuë discards her velvet robe. Her body gleams in the starlight and her arms wreath about you. She offers to you the priceless gift of herself, the gift that even in the land of fairy may only be given once. It is something you have longed for but for which you feared to ask, but now it is given with love and a promise to wait until Merlin shall walk again in Tir-nan-Og.

The only sounds are those of the nightbirds and the small sighs and whispered words that pass between lovers at such times. The grass is cool to your bodies and the tiny flowers beneath Nimuë's body give up their perfume in an ecstasy that matches hers. For her sake you try to be as gentle as you can but the tide that overtakes you both is too great a force to be denied for long and all too soon it recedes, leaving you entwined in each other's arms.

In a while you stir and look down at Nimuë as she sleeps with a little smile upon her lips, her graceful limbs relaxed in the aftermath of love. Gently so as not to disturb her dreaming, you take one of the roses from her hair and catch upon its white petals the red drops of her maiden blood. Rising, you move to stand in the starlight and summoning your magical powers, fashion from that light a gleaming crystal in the form of a heart. Within it you enclose the rose and its precious contents.

You dress quickly, for by dawn you must be in the Land of Albion ready to begin the task of arranging the birth of Arthur, the High King. Wrapped warmly in your cloak you carry the sleeping Nimuë in your arms through the garden and back into the castle. All is now quiet but in the empty hall stands Aengus and beside him your mother. They understand that you do not want to say goodbye to Nimuë, but will leave quietly while she sleeps. Aengus takes her from you. You know they will love her and guard her well. To your mother you give the crystal heart with instructions to place it upon Nimuë's pillow. You kiss her once and then your mother, place a hand on your father's shoulder and it is time to leave.

One of your teachers waits to take you to the place of departure. All that goes with you is a staff made of hawthorn topped with a crystal that once lay on the breast of the Priest of the Sun in Atlantis and, in a leather pouch about your neck, a lock of dark silky hair that smells of roses. You wait as your companion draws the two worlds together and slowly a door opens between them.

You see a forest and an arch of hawthorn bushes, and just beyond a gnarled and ancient oak tree that will be your signpost when you need to find the way back. A quick farewell and you pass through into Albion and the door closes behind you. With the power of the crystal you burn a secret symbol into the trunk of the tree to mark its significance and then you turn mind, will and body towards your task. But your heart you have left far behind sleeping in a fairy castle.

# Ritual 5

# THE RAISING OF OSIRIS

## The Programme

The story of Osiris is probably the best known myth in the western world and it comes in several versions. The basic format, for those who have little knowledge of Egyptian mythology, concerns the ongoing battle between good and evil and begins with the birth of two sets of twins to the Star Goddess Nuit by her brother Geb the Earth God. Osiris and Isis were the firstborn, the bright twins destined to be man and wife, king and queen of the land of Egypt, Gods who descended to earth to bring the concept of agriculture and settlement to humanity. The second set of twins were Nepthys and Set, the dark chthonic or under the earth God forms.

The Gods planned that each set of twins would rule in their appointed ways and places, but even the Gods cannot escape the occasional disruption of their plans. Set grew violently jealous of his brother and opposed him in every possible way, culminating in the murder of Osiris. Here the legend becomes less clear with many differing versions, but foremost among them is one telling of the body of Osiris being torn into 14 pieces. This rending of the body of a God-king is widespread throughout world traditions and information can be found in the chapters on The Sacrificed God in Frazer's book *The Golden Bough*.

Prior to the murder Nephthys had borne a son, Anubis, to her brother Osiris, with the consent of Isis who had, as yet, no children. Isis took the young prince and brought him up as her own, teaching him all her magical ways and bringing him to full power as a magician and, even more important, as a Walker between the Worlds, one who was able to exist in the underworld, the physical world and the upper world.

After the death of Osiris and the scattering of his body Set usurped the throne and ruled in his stead. Isis disguised herself and with Anubis roamed the land for many years, searching for

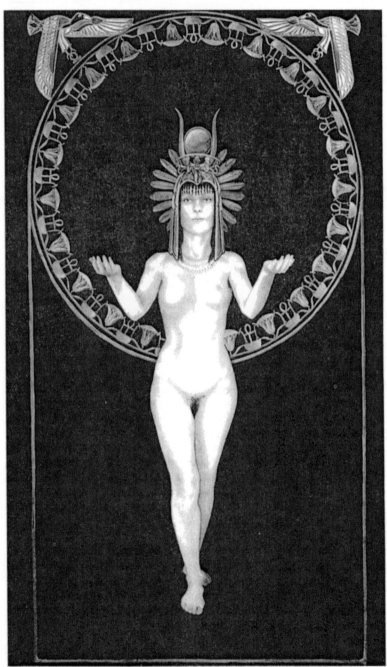

*Figure 14:* Isis *(Paul Hardy)*

each part of her husband's body until she had them all, all that is save for the phallus, which legend tells us was eaten by a fish. At her temple on the island of Philae she gathered the dismembered body together and with the help of Anubis not only made them whole but brought new life to the dead God-king. The missing phallus she replaced with one made of gold, albeit it gold made into living flesh by her magical powers. By this means she succeeded in impregnating herself with the child Horus, later called 'the Avenger' when he overthrew Set.

This myth sets the scene for the ritual and its sphere on the Tree is that of Tiphereth, the sphere of harmony, balance and sacrifice. The ritual itself owes its basic form to one far more ancient referring to the conception of Horus. In this present format it is seen as a balance between the male power of sacrifice and regeneration, symbolized by the softening of the penis after intercourse and its recovery when desire once more stimulates its new growth, and the female power of life and death through the process of birth. Thus the intention of the ritual is to bring increased harmony and balance to the relationship of the two people taking part. The 'Horus child' that is conceived is an emotional, mental and spiritual concept and not a physical child – the ritual for calling a soul into incarnation can be found in the sphere of Binah.

The main accessory for this ritual is a life-sized outline of the male partner, Osiris. For this you will need several rolls of strong brown wrapping paper. Lay out on the floor two or, if needed, three lengths of the paper as this may need taping together with clear tape to give the width. The man then lies down on the paper while his partner draws the outline of his body on it with a thick black marker pen. When this is done the resulting outline must be cut into 13 pieces as in Fig 15. The fourteenth piece is of course the missing phallus and testicles: these are drawn separately from the main outline in gold foil. You now have the dismembered body of Osiris. You can use cloth if you wish to make something more permanent that can be used again.

Ideally the catafalque for the body of Osiris would be a single bed draped with a white sheet scattered with flower heads and petals. If this is not possible then use the bottom end of a double bed covered in the same way. About three or four feet in front of the bed place a small table to act as an altar and cover it with a white or blue cloth. On this place a small bowl of warm scented water with flower petals and sweet herbs in it, a small cloth to bathe the body of Osiris and a larger one of soft absorbent material (not a towel), with which to dry him, some massage oil, scented or not as you wish, and an Ankh of any size or type. In addition you will need a small glass of wine and an Egyptian collar (see Fig

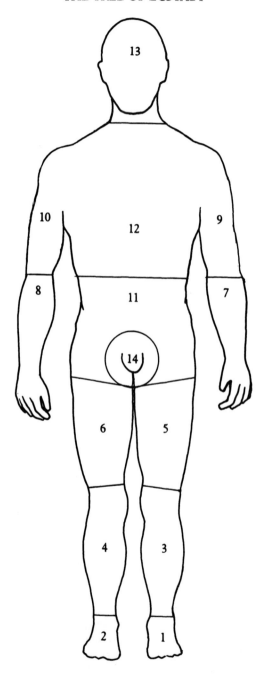

*Figure 15:* The dismembered body of Osiris

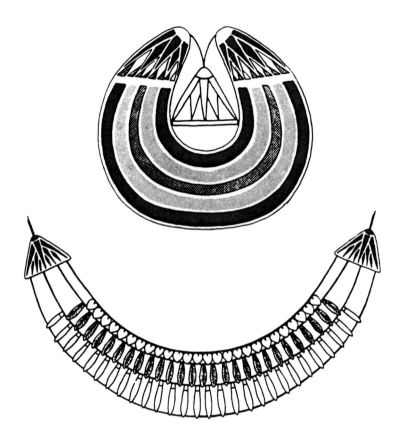

*Figure 16:* An Egyptian collar

16). If you want to extend the dressing of the king's body, then the Red Crown of Egypt is easily made from red cartridge paper or card. The golden phallus is symbolized by a penis sheath made of gold material and fitted to cover it when fully erect. Osiris wears the collar, head-dress and sheath, and waits quietly in a corner of the room until Isis has reassembled the body.

Isis wears a white robe opening fully down the front, made of any semi-transparent lightweight material, with a golden cord around her waist and a collar like that of Osiris and perhaps golden sandals if she wishes. Bracelets pushed high up the arm, ear-rings and a golden ribbon tied around the forehead will complete her costume.

The room may be decorated with anything you have that might add to the atmosphere, for example tall vases with flowers or branches, coloured silk scarves as hangings or drapes, and statues/pictures in the Egyptian style. The ritual itself *must* be memorized to obtain the full effect. The pieces of Osiris' body must be scattered about the room or the adjoining room. Incense could be a good quality Kyphi, and must be used in two burners, one each at the head and feet of Osiris.

Now we come to the exercises for this ritual. Please do not forget the need for complete celibacy during the week preceding the rite.

First the exercises for the woman: on rising stretch upwards as fully as possible letting the arms pull you up until you are standing on your toes and fully extended, then let your body come down gently and allow it to slump over until your arms hang down to the floor. Now stand up, slowly curving your back, vertebra by vertebra. Now, for the second part, sit either in the Lotus position or the more usual western style of the God form. Back erect, visualize a golden Lotus above the head pouring out a liquid light. Feel it fill the top part of your head and seep down into the pineal centre. Hold the light there until you can feel the centre begin to pulsate under the stimulation of the liquid. Now allow it to flow down into the throat centre and hold it again. Wait until you feel the throat begin to throb and then pass it through into the heart centre. Hold it steady and allow the light to pass into the bloodstream so that it passes around the body. Feel the glow as it passes through one organ after another and fills them with strength and power. Allow five minutes for this and then pull the light back into the heart centre and withdraw it. Follow this exactly for the first two days, then on the third and fourth days pull the light down to the solar centre and send it flowing over the entire skin surface of the body, enriching, cleansing and revitalizing it. Then withdraw as before. On the fifth and sixth days take the light down to the genital centre, touch the tip of the tongue to the roof of the mouth and allow the light to follow the meridians centred on the perineum, one running up the spinal column over the head to the roof of the mouth, the other up the front of the body to the tip of the tongue. After five minutes withdraw and close as usual.

The evening exercise is also done together, either nude or robed as you please. Face each other and place the palms of the hands together. Picture the golden Lotus over the head as in the morning exercise and allow its light to flow down as before into the heart centre. At this point the man flows it out down the right arm into his right hand on into the woman's left hand, up her arm and into the heart centre. She flows her power down her right arm into the right hand and into the man's left hand, up the arm and into his heart centre. This establishes a flow of energy and male/female power through both bodies. Do this for a period of three minutes.

For the second part of the evening exercise, the woman turns her back to the man who presses close to her so that their bodies are touching from shoulder to knee. The woman places her hands in the age-old gesture of concealment, one hand across her breasts and the other covering the genitals. (This gesture is one of summoning the power to the emotional and creative centres rather than one of concealment.) The man puts his arms around the woman and with one hand covers the solar centre in a protective gesture, and with the other covers the sacred centre of the womb.

At this point the woman summons her 'Isis' power in the form of a silver star. It starts above the head and is pulled down through the crown, pineal and throat centres and down to the genitals where it rests, flooding the area with power. A second star is brought down in the same way and placed in the sacred centre of the womb, then a third is stored in the solar centre. The fourth is placed in the heart, then one each in the throat, pineal centre and just below the crown centre. Now the woman empowers the star symbols and the man links himself to each star with the exception of the sacred centre, which is for the woman alone. The power will ricochet from one to the other all the way up. It must be visualized as a silver thread that bursts into fire at each centre point. Keep it going, empowering the thread from the genital centre and joining it finally at the emergence point. Do this for no more than five minutes, ending with the man retaining each star burst as it hits the centres so that he ends the week with a radiant star empowering each centre.

If you are not familiar with the Egyptian Tradition then it is important to read up on as much of the subject as you can before attempting the ritual. Be prepared for emotional and mental pressure during it, and for a varying intensity of after-effects. The man should be aware of the great love and pride of Osiris for his sister wife and the magical 'pull' as she reassembles the body. Then, as she prepares to recall life into the dead God-king, he must feel the energy beginning to pulse in each centre by visualizing the power stars left in his body by the evening exercise. Meditation on the symbols of the Ankh, the Lotus, the Djed and the Tet will help to stabilize the power centres after the ritual. As usual ensure your privacy and prepare everything beforehand. If possible this ritual is best done just before dawn so that Osiris rises with the sun.

# The Raising of Osiris

## Sphere = Tiphereth. Keynote = Harmony and Unity Through Love.

*The ritual begins with the lamentation of Isis for her husband. She stands before the prepared bier, draws the mourning veil over her head and kneels down in the mourning attitude with one hand on her breast and the other arm and hand raised and curved over her head.*

*Isis:* Weep, weep, O ye lands of the south, for Osiris my love has gone down into the darkness of death. Mourn, mourn, ye lands of the west for his like shall not come again for a thousand years. Cry aloud, O ye lands of the north, with your cold winds freeze the heart of Isis that she may feel no more pain. Alas, ye lands of the east for no longer does the light of Osiris shine forth to welcome the dawn. My eyes behold him no more and my arms are empty.

*She stands up and raises her arms up.*

Gods of Egypt, I call on thee for help. To thee, Ptah, Lord of Life, I call for the power to raise my beloved from the sleep of death for one day and one night.

*She turns to the left.*

Khnum, upon whose wheel the clay of life is moulded, fashion me a son like a warrior of Ra.

*She turns to the right.*

Min, Lord of Fertility, breathe life into the sun child of Isis and Osiris.

*She turns her back to the bier.*

Nuit, my starborn mother, with thy power I will blend my own and Osiris shall live again. Atum Ra, Lord of the Gods, grant me my desire, and release the spirit of Osiris from the underworld.

*She turns to face the bier and bows, then lights the two incense burners and fills them with kyphi. With the first one she censes the place where the body will lie, then replaces it at the head. With the second she censes the area where she will work, then places it at the foot.*

*Now, one by one, she collects each piece of the body and puts them in place: first the two feet and then the lower legs, the upper legs, the lower torso, the upper torso, the lower arms and hands, the upper arms and hands, and finally the head. As she brings each piece she censes it with each censer alternately. There is a speech for each one.*

*Isis:* Every part of thy body have I found and restored, my love, all save for the rod of life and that I shall create anew from the gold of the sun, symbol of life.

*right foot:*
Let thy right foot be placed upon the earth in gladness.

*left foot:*
Let thy left foot be placed upon the earth in power.
*right lower leg:*
Let thy right knee kneel before the Gods in prayer.
*left lower leg:*
Let thy left knee kneel before the Gods in suppliance.
*right upper leg:*
Let thy right thigh be as strong as a tree.
*left upper leg:*
Let thy left thigh be as straight as a measuring rod.
*phallus:*
Let thy rod of life be potent in its strength.
*lower torso:*
Let thy lower body be strong in its manhood.
*upper torso:*
Let thy upper body be royal in its appearance.
*right lower arm:*
Let they right hand wield the flail of justice.
*left lower arm:*
Let thy left hand hold the crook of mercy.
*right upper arm:*
Let thy right shoulder bear the weight of rule.
*left upper arm:*
Let thy left shoulder shelter the head of Isis.
*head:*
Let thy head wear the royal crown, thy mouth know breath, thy nostrils
    smell incense, thine ears hear my voice. Open thine eyes to me, O my
    beloved.

*The whole body should now be assembled. During this time Osiris stands
ready in a corner of the room, waiting for the summons. As Isis speaks he
draws nearer, and when Isis closes her eyes and speaks the great invocation
he lies down on the outline, crosses his arms over the breast and closes his
eyes.*

   *Isis:* Spirit of Osiris, draw near and harken to the words of thy
wife and queen. To thy right stands Ptah, Lord of Life and to thy
left Khnum, the God of Form. Before thee stands our mother Nuit,
mighty in her strength, and behind thee stands Atum Ra, the
Creator of All Things. I, Isis, have interceded for thee, for a day
and a night to be returned to me. Within that time we shall create
a child of mind and spirit. From Isis and Osiris shall come a
harmony of peace and beauty to cover the world with its glory.
From the two shall come the one, the mighty new aeon that will
be the guardian of the Earth Mother.

   *By now Osiris is standing at the head of the bier ready to assume the
form of life. As Isis begins the next speech he lies down on the marked
bier.*

   *Isis:* Live, Osiris, live, lord of the land of Khem, live my beloved and lie in my arms. Breathe from the sacred Ankh of Ptah, draw substance from the hands of Khnum, be born again from thy mother Nuit, and live by the will of Atum Ra. I, Isis, Queen of Heaven, summon the powers of the Gods of Egypt and cause the heart of Osiris to beat again.

*She places her hands over his heart and then passes them over and down the whole body.*

Return, lord of thy people, return and live.

*Osiris breathes deeply, lifting the rib cage high at each breath. Isis leans over him and kisses him. His eyes remain closed; he lies still. Now Isis takes water and bathes his body gently, including the face, then dries him with the soft cloth.*

Isis: With water from the Nile I bathe thee. Like the river thou shalt rise and flood the land.

*She now takes the oil and rubs it into his flesh, lightly over the arms, legs and body, more strongly, and well diluted with non-scented oil, on the phallus, continuing until Osiris is fully erect. He should assist her by using visualization and allowing the power of the ritual to maintain full erection.*

Isis: With precious oils from the south I anoint thee and cause the arrow of Osiris to spring from the bow of his body.

*She takes the oil and rubs a little into each armpit, onto the breastbone and on either side of the scrotum.*

With the unguent of sexual power do I touch thee and make thee potent in thy rising.

*She dips her finger in the wine and touches his lips, then holds the Ankh to his mouth.*

With wine and the symbol of life I open thy mouth. Waken to me, my beloved.

*Osiris opens his eyes.*

Osiris: Sister, queen and wife, I rejoice in the sight of thee. I was lost in the darkness and thy voice has called me to life. I spoke with the Gods and have walked in their ways. When I go forth again I shall walk in the light and be one with them. Thou art my love, sweet singer of songs, Isis of the gentle voice and loving hands. Behold thou art beautiful in my sight. Thy breasts are like doves that come to me when called, thy belly is a curve of ivory and thy thighs are like the slender reeds that line the Nile banks. Dark and mysterious is thy cave of stars wherein the pleasure and joy of Osiris can be found. Thy feet are like small fishes that glide through quiet water. In thee I find rest and tranquillity, strength and wisdom. One short day and night with thee then I must return to Amenti. Come, join with me and let my arrow fly to thy heart.

*Isis undoes her waist cord and lets fall her robe then removes the penis sheath from Osiris. Again she caresses him and ensures his erection, then she stands over him on the bier, straddling his body and, holding her arms crossed over her breast, she visualizes the star empowerment of her body centres as in the evening exercise. Then she kneels above him and slowly lowers her body until the phallus just touches her body.*

*Osiris:* Open the cave of stars to thy love. Let us invoke the gift of Hathor, the Goddess of love. Pour out thy honeyed sweetness and accept my offering in its place.

*He touches her breasts, belly and clitoris.*

We are twice born in the world of the Gods and in the world of men. Mighty art thou, Isis, for even the rod of life rises to thee and bows in supplication.

*He brings her down until he is fully sheathed in her.*

Great Isis, mistress of magic, to the Gods is my joy given in honour.

*Isis:* My love and lord, king and brother, thou are the Nile in flood and I am the fields of Ra. To thee, Nuit, lady of stars, mother of all things, to thee my joy in honour.

*The mating proceeds to its conclusion but the power of it is offered in silent worship to the Gods. Isis sinks down upon the breast of Osiris and they rest and visualize the 'child' of the rite, the harmony and peace of the world. See in the mind's eye a Lotus bud which gradually opens, emitting a brilliant light. Seated in its heart is a golden child, its finger to its lips in the ancient sign of silence, the sign of the initiate. The child rises and grows brighter until it can no longer be seen, for it has become one with the aura of the earth itself. If it is desired by both, a second mating may be enjoyed for its own pleasure. Then both should bathe and eat before closing down.*

# The Pathworking

Visualize a running river. On either side the narrow fields that edge the sacred Nile soon give way to barren redstone cliffs and stunted palms. The large island in the middle of the river looms darkly, only the very tops of the trees catching the moon's light. A small shallow boat is moving slowly towards it and we can dimly see the outline of two passengers and a larger, more solid outline. The oarsman brings the boat close in to the shore and we hear the scrape of it on the stones as it is beached. One of the passengers rises, a tall, broad-shouldered young man who moves with grace and strength. He helps the second figure from the boat. Smaller and lighter, this is obviously a woman wrapped in a cloak and veiled against prying eyes.

The boatman and the younger man lift the boat's cargo ashore and carry it inland, and the woman follows. Ahead gleams the white stone of a small temple and there on the altar stone within its ruins the two men gently place their burden, a large wooden box wrapped in cloth. The boatman stands up, eases his back, then turns to the woman and kneels to her, lifting the hem of her robe to his lips. Rising, he turns to the young man and bows deeply, placing his work-worn hands between those of the younger man as if in fealty. He refuses the gold that is offered, accepting only the blessing that the woman gives him, then he returns to the boat and rows away.

Isis removes her heavy cloak and walks to the covered sarcophagus that contains the body of her beloved husband and king, Osiris. She places a long narrow hand on it, gently, as if touching the man within. Then she stands back and bids her foster son Anubis unwrap the box. When revealed it is seen to be covered in paintings and inlaid work of great skill. Time has darkened the paint and many of the precious stones are missing, but it is still beautiful. Anubis opens his father's coffin with his sword and as the moon clears the trees its light falls on the face of the man lying within. His face is unmarked by decay: it is as if he were asleep so calm are his features.

Anubis lifts his father's body from its prison and pushes the empty sarcophagus aside. Osiris is then laid on the altar top and Isis throws herself weeping on his breast, kissing the cold lips and murmuring the love words she used of old. Anubis waits awhile then gently coaxes her away to sit on a stone seat while he fetches water from the river and washes the body clean of the accumulated dust and dirt of 10 years. Then he brings to Isis a second bundle left by the boatman and from it she brings the royal robes and regalia that Osiris wore when he lived.

Together they dress the dead God-king in his robes and place the crown on his head and the crook and flail in his hands. Then Anubis steps backs and begins to pace around the little temple and as he does so there begins to build up a great ring of light. It has many colours that glitter and gleam in the moonlight and soon the whole temple is encased within its protection.

Isis moves to the head of Osiris and begins to invoke the great Gods of Egypt. Soon their mighty forms appear behind her. She passes her power to Anubis and he takes his place on the left side of the body and invokes the second company of Gods. Isis moves then to the feet of Osiris, again her voice rings through the stillness of the night and soon the Goddesses come into manifestation behind her. Now Anubis comes to the right side of the body and calls the mighty assessors to witness the plan of Isis.

Now a great ring of Godlike beings surround Osiris and fill the temple with their power. Isis goes to each one in turn asking for their help in restoring her loved one to life. As she finishes her plea there is silence, and in that silence the Gods confer. Anubis comforts his foster mother as the moon rises to its zenith and begins its downward journey. Then Ptah, the God of life, steps forward.

He commends Isis and Anubis for their devotion and for the work that both Isis and Osiris have done for the people of earth, but the complete return of life to the dead king is not to be. But the Gods will allow him one day and one night of life and during that time a son will be conceived who will avenge his father's death at the hands of Set the usurper. To provide the life force needed they must take from Anubis one day and one night of his life and give it to Osiris. To this Anubis agrees, and Ptah sinks his hand into the breast of the young man. When he withdraws it a shimmering pearl of light gleams in his fingers. The God moves to the body of Osiris and places the pearl of life deep in his breast. Each of the Gods passes by the bier and Isis and Anubis standing at the head and feet of the king. As they pass they bless them and disappear into the darkness beyond the temple.

Motionless at their posts the two guardians wait. The long night moves to its close, the moon slips gently down towards the horizon and the sky begins to lighten. The gates of dawn swing open to herald the appearance of Ra's sun boat, and as it tips the hills we hear a sound in the temple, the sound of breathing. The breast of Osiris lifts and the colour returns to his face. Hardly daring to hope, Isis moves to his side and bends over him, then flings back her head and cries out with joy and gladness, 'He lives, he lives, Osiris lives and breathes!'

Anubis comes with her cloak to wrap her against the morning chill and stands with her as the eyes that have been closed for so long open and look up at them. For a moment Osiris can see nothing, then the faces of his loved ones become clear to him and a smile breaks over his face. He is helped to his feet and embraces his wife who has never ceased to search for his body or wavered in her determination to wrest him back from the dead. Osiris knows he does not have much time but he is content with what has been given and knows also that he owes this space of time to the son who has given him 24 hours of his own lifetime that he may be with Isis.

Anubis withdraws and leaves the lovers together. They wander down to the edge of the river and begin their time together. Short as it is, it will be enough for them – more than they expected to have. The gold and silver of royalty are stripped away and rather than a king and his queen it is a man and woman that blend with the shadows and become one shadow that moves in sensuous joy beneath the trees.

# Ritual 6

# THE TWO OF SWORDS

## The Programme

It is unpleasant to have to admit it, but violence can be sexually stimulating to some kinds of people. But it must be understood that *violence has no place in sex magic* despite the nastier type of video, pornographic magazines and the tabloid press. However, what can be termed 'sexual banter' is part of a whole chain of behaviour that starts between boys and girls at school and continues into adulthood. In primitive tribes the exchange of humorous insults between the sexes is considered to be a part of any big celebration. Where sexual magic is concerned, and in this next ritual in particular, violence is really not the correct term to use, nor is aggression, but perhaps 'a loving struggle' comes close to it. For many women the very word 'violence' carries with it memories of pain, humiliation and low self-esteem and should never be used to describe behaviour in any ritual, let alone one where sexual power is part of the work.

During our teenage years and right into the early years of marriage rough and tumble, retreat and chase, capture and claiming is a very real part of love and sex. The 16-year-old boys' teasing of their female classmates, the girls' lofty disdain and ignoring of their clumsy attempts at sexual advances – often subconscious on the boys' part – are all practice and a polishing of sexual skills. When the teenagers are older and a mate is being seriously sought, the whole gamut is gone through again, but with more intent and with an end in view. In the early, euphoric days of marriage a couple will often indulge in games that end up in a loving romp and a struggle for supremacy, games which neither is serious about winning, only about the promise of a heightened sexual response and its outcome.

In ritual this can be taken into the realms of the knight and the warrior maid, and these will be the archetypes used in the rite of

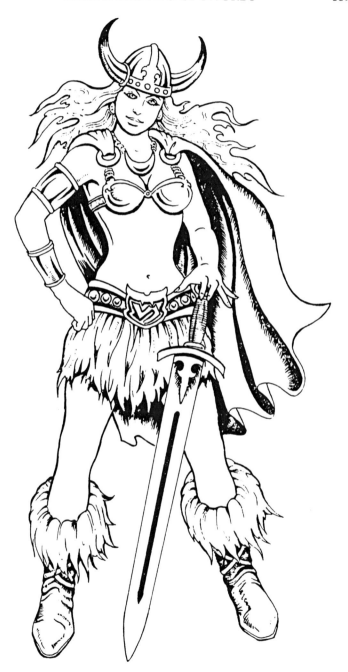

*Figure 17:* The Warrior Maid

the Two of Swords. I make no apology here for blatantly drawing on every sword and sorcery and fantasy novel ever written! In fact this ritual might well be described as magical fun with a sexual flavour, and before this raises more eyebrows than have already been stretched to the limit in this book, let me say this. If one cannot laugh and even make a little gentle fun of one's religion, then there is something wrong with both you and the religion.

There are many ways to look at the archetype of the knight, from the gentle and rather insipid Galahad to his father, the gallant but luckless Lancelot, from the bloodthirsty Teutonic knights converting by the sword to the idealized figure of St George, with variations all the way along. The idea is enshrined in the idiom of our language as 'the white knight on a charger' or 'a knight in shining armour' – something most ladies dream of at some point in their lives. King Arthur is seen as the perfect royal knight and small boys dream of being a Knight of the Round Table – and not only small boys either, much larger boys are just as given to dreaming.

The legendary hero also comes into the category of 'the knight'. He leaves the family home and goes seeking for the ultimate treasure. This treasure may be a grail, a magic carpet, a flying horse, an island with buried treasure or the heart of a sleeping princess. For both sexes fairy tales often provide our first templates for dream archetypes. At first it is the fairy queen and Cinderella, Robin Hood and Peter Pan, then later on it is the latest rock or film star. We learn the art of fantasy and day-dreaming at an early age and it never leaves us, though in some people it gets buried very deeply.

The warrior maid archetype, although an ancient one, has only really come into her own during the last 20 years or so. The modern version is very much a product of the female revolution. Women everywhere are proving that they can do almost every job a man does just as well and sometimes better. As always in every revolution there is a tendency for things to swing too far at first and an imbalance results until things settle down. We are coming up to this point as we enter the last decade of the twentieth century.

As examples of the warrior maid we might start with Diana the huntress and Athene the Greek Goddess of wisdom and include Sekhmet, the lion-headed Goddess of Egypt sometimes called the Sword or Arm of Ra, the fierce Valkyries, the battlemaids of Norse mythology, and the British warrior maid Boudicca, Queen of the Iceni. Hyppolyta, Queen of the Amazons, led her female warriors against the finest of the Greek armies, and there are tales in Irish mythology of women who fought in battle alongside their menfolk as indeed did the women of the Samurai families in ancient Japan.

There is no dearth of examples and if one looks closely at them it will be seen that warriors notwithstanding, they were still very feminine women and much courted by the warriors and heroes of their time.

Just as there are options open to men in the way they live their lives, so there are options open to women. For some the exacting task of being a wife, mother and Priestess of the Hearthfire is still the one they prefer. For others the professional life offers more. It is recognized now that not all women are born with a mothering instinct and some have little or no wish to bear children. They follow the path of Diana and Athene and prefer to remain free. Yet others will choose the best of both worlds, rising to the top of their chosen profession and then, when they feel they have fulfilled themselves in that field, they will marry comparatively late in life and even raise a family in their forties. It is no longer a stigma to be unmarried in your thirties and to prefer a modern apartment and a good car to marriage and children. The warrior maid has won back her right to be as free as she wants to be.

In the strict sense of the word, the Two of Swords is not a ritual, it is a magical encounter between equals. There are many instances when events not normally considered to be a ritual take on a ritualistic quality because the way in which they are enacted becomes an 'intention'. This is seen in the martial arts, especially in the area of sword play, in the slow and stately movements of T'ai Chi, and in the flowing exercises of a ballet dancer at the barre. Anything done consistently and with intention becomes a ritual on its own level. The traditional Sunday roast with beef, Yorkshire pudding and two vegetables, and a doze in the afternoon under the guise of reading the papers is a ritual performed every weekend in countless homes in Britain, so is the Fourth of July parade in America. Humans make rituals out of almost every aspect of life. This 'magical encounter' is ritualistic in its pattern of intention, which is to decide the winner in a battle of wits, magic and sexual stamina. It has a sexual content and for the first time in the book, the pleasure is yours to enjoy.

In ancient Sparta both boys and girls were trained as athletes and expected to compete in annual games. They trained, slept and ate under strict discipline and with little comfort in their surroundings The very word 'spartan' has now come to mean bare and joyless surroundings. The character of the warrior maid in the modern fantasy paperbacks could well have been modelled on the girls of Sparta: she is slender but strong, skilled in the use of weapons, can ride for days without getting saddle-sore, wears next to nothing and seems impervious to cold, hunger and ill treatment. However she, like the Mountie, always gets her man. In every partnership there should be time and space for fun and if it can include a little 'loving aggression' all the better. I might add that in this particular battle there is no guaranteed winner – either one of you may win, you may both lose or both succeed.

Like the third ritual this one goes on all day and comes in three parts. One is physical, one is mental, the other is . . . interesting. In the first two you have a choice of venue and 'weapons', in the other – well, let us say that all is fair in love and war.

As in all magical encounters there is a prize. It should be unusual, beautiful and of course full of magical power. My suggestion is that long before you reach this particular ritual you select a suitable object, say a medallion of unusual design with a stone set at the centre. If funds will run to it, have it made to your own design and share the cost. This will be the jewel you both seek and will be ritually consecrated and empowered at the beginning of the week leading up to the 'battle'. A challenge must be issued and accepted with the magical jewel as the prize and a third party appointed as the keeper of the jewel. The actual challenge must be issued on the morning of the chosen day.

Let us look at the physical test first and at the selection of weapons you may use. Real swords are out of the question unless you happen to fence. But if you cannot use swords, you can use Batacas. These are soft cloth-covered bats made from plastic foam. They are easily made at home, or you may be able to get them from a martial arts shop. There is no way you can hurt each other, even using all your strength and they make ideal 'weapons' for a rough and tumble – a bit like pillow fighting really. If you decide to use the Batacas then I suggest you do it early in the morning before breakfast. It works up an appetite and clears the air for the rest of the day. All aggression is swept away and the shared laughter is marvellous. A word of warning: the night before please clear away all small ornaments, valuables, pictures and anything that might get broken. A Bataca battle may start on the bed but it will gradually range over the whole room and possibly further afield. Try to outwit each other by being the first to wake up and start the battle. (By the way this kind of fighting raises the libido sky high, but I am afraid the rule of no sex holds until the *last* phase of the day. Think of it as *hors d'oeuvres* before the feast.)

Your alternative weapon to the Batacas is competitiveness: running, swimming, badminton, squash, anything that offers a fair game on either side. Male partners can be handicapped if longer legs or physical strength offer too great an advantage. The whole object is to outdo or outlast each other and get pleasantly tired doing so.

The second part, the mental 'battle', may need some preparation on both sides. If you both play chess, that is good since the battle can be decided by the winning of a game. A better game – because it is even harder – is that of Wei Chi. Its devotees claim that it is even older than chess, and it is certainly more devious and well suited to the 'off the wall logic' some women have brought to a fine art. (You may find it difficult to obtain, but try shops run by native Chinese or carrying Chinese goods.) You might also try poker, backgammon or any game involving mental skill. If preferred you might like to make this 'battle' a contest of mental agility and buy a book of Mensa questions and puzzles and challenge each other in that way. Whatever way you choose to do it, the outcome is important. If one person has won both times, no matter which sex, they get to plan the layout for the final phase. If it works out at one all, then the keeper of the jewel must come up with three questions. Two out of three correct answers will name the winner.

The final phase has several options for its planner. What you will need for it depends on what you intend doing! Your essential ingredient is darkness inside the house. Draw every curtain, clear all unnecessary furniture and anything that might drop, crash, break or stub a toe out of the way. It is best to have a light snack about half-past four or five o'clock as you are not going to eat until late. The kitchen is out of bounds once you have prepared a meal, set the oven timer or put the food into the fridge, and set the wine to either 'breathe' or cool according to type.

The losing partner must be sent from the house while it is being prepared. But no going to the local pub and forgetting to be back at the time agreed, or you may find the Batacas have been swapped for something a lot harder! You will also forfeit the prize. While the other person is away the opponent may begin to lay down his or her web.

With a ball of thick twine lay down a path for your partner to follow by touch alone. Make it as tortuous as you can, leading back and forth through as many of the rooms as you think you will need to make it a good hard test. Try giving your opponent different floor coverings in unexpected places, such as a square of cushions where they least expect it, or a rough matting where there is normally a smooth floor. If you really want to surprise them, try putting a few potato crisps at strategic points! It is surprising how loud the crunch will sound in a quiet and darkened house. All the while they must keep hold of the cord and follow where it leads. A warning here: *never* put down anything that can cause your partner to slip, trip up or fall over. Do not polish under mats, and make sure that though they follow the cord, there is no danger of injuring themselves. Do not on any account use the thread to lead a person *downstairs* – upstairs, yes, but *never* the other way, for in the dark, and expecting something to happen at any moment when they are already jumpy, you may cause a fall or serious injury. This is a battle of wits, a game between lovers, not all-out war!

For this last phase you have a choice: you can become the warrior maid or knight proper, in which case the thread can lead your partner to a place cleared for a last battle – and you can decide if you are going to give in gracefully or fight to win – or the thread can lead your partner right into a scene with everything laid out for a loving seduction, which the other must try to avoid. There are more ways to win a battle than with swords! Oh, by the way, did I mention that the one following the thread must undress once inside the door and follow it naked?!

There are all sorts of possibilities here – for instance you might decide to tie a small bell to the thread somewhere along the line. You know where they are, but they have no idea where you are. (Think of it along the lines of the running battles between Inspector Clouseau of *Pink Panther* fame and his maniac man servant Cato.) A nice touch is a towel soaked in iced water and laid across a doorway – it can be a real shocker. Fine cotton threads suspended from the lintel will feel like spider webs in the dark. If you feel you *should* give them a small advantage you can allow them a box with just three matches in it . . .

There must be an agreement as to just where the seeker will be able to find the first end of the thread. No cheating here, and use of torches or lights is not allowed. If you are using the warrior maid/knight fantasy then both should wear a token on a ribbon round the arm or waist. Once this is taken the battle is over. Please note you do not wear the ribbon around your neck, for in the heat of battle you can cause injury to your partner. Play fair: once your token has been taken, surrender. (It is sometimes more fun.) Knights, temper your strength to your opponent if she is five foot two and you are six foot, and remember a woman's breasts bruise easily. Warrior maids, there are some things not meant to be grabbed and twisted – take care, you want to conquer not incapacitate!

The rules must be made quite clear from the start: no biting, scratching, or use of pain to subdue in any way. This goes as much for the warrior maids as for the knights, and applies equally to all three sessions. Once the victor has carried the day he or she is entitled to the magical jewel *and the loser*. Now is the time to set your sexuality free and share its power with your partner. Seek out the jewel and place it between you as close as possible to the point of joining as you make love: it will enhance its power a hundredfold.

The day has been filled with excitement, struggle and antici-pation and the joy of sharing your strength with one you love and respect. Many people are afraid of Geburah, and see it as the sphere of destruction and death. I have tried in this ritual encounter to show that sometimes all that is destroyed are subconscious fears, grudges, resentments and the niggling doubts that beset any partnership, even the best. In this Geburic situation the only death is the 'little death', *le petit mort*, of the sexual climax.

There are no exercises for this month's ritual – you will have enough exercise keeping up with the preparations. There is a certain kind of bond that comes into being between 'warriors'. It thrives on shared excitement, a little danger and a lot of togetherness. The sphere of Geburah can be a very worthwhile experience, the more so because you probably did not expect this particular sphere to be one of fun and laughter. If you intend to use body oils, make them unscented, for you can be found in the dark by a scent. For an alternative incense try this: yohimbe 3/4, ginger 1/4, damiana 1/2, cinnamon 1/2 mixed with ambergris oil and a little water. If nothing else it should be an interesting evening!

# The Consecration Ritual for the Magical Jewel

## Sphere = Geburah. Keynote = The Combat between Beauty and Strength.

*This ritual is for four people: the warrior maid in the north, the knight of the sun in the south, the keeper of the jewel in the east and the priestess of the jewel in the west. You will therefore need the help of two friends for this consecration ritual. The maid and the knight should each have a sword or an athame-type dagger to represent a sword. East and West should be robed. The maid might wear a leotard with a cloak and a wide belt to carry her sword, plain boots if she has them, and a black or green ribbon forehead band. The knight may be barechested and may wear plain trousers tucked into boots if available, a cloak, a belt and sword. The altar is covered by a white cloth and carries a chalice in the west in which the jewel has been placed overnight covered by water. In the north is a dish of salt, in the east is a censer with incense already burning and in the south a short but thick candle either red or yellow in colour. The four take their places.*

*The keeper paces three times around the altar.*

*Keeper:* Within the sacred circle safe from all harm we come to consecrate the magical jewel of Shemataka. With this jewel a man or a woman may aspire to be the high priest or priestess of the earth herself, with the power to ease the planet's wounds and bring peace to the internal heart of the Great Mother. Priestess of the jewel, bring forth the Eye of Shemataka.

*The priestess takes the jewel from the water and gives it to the keeper.*

*Priestess:* Into thy hands, master of magic, I place the Eye of Shemataka to be consecrated and made holy.

*The keeper takes the jewel and holds it in the rising smoke of the incense.*

*Keeper:* In the name of Shemataka, the Goddess of the deep inner earth where all precious stones are born in fire, I bless and make pure this jewel. I open the heart of this stone and place within a star *(makes gesture of catching a star and placing it in the stone)* that it may light the way of its wearer through the darkest night, in the darkest hour.

*He hands the jewel to the priestess. She sprinkles it with water from the chalice.*

*Priestess:* In the name of Thetis, Goddess of the deep, I bless and make pure this precious stone. Within its heart I will place a single drop of the ocean of space *(makes gesture of putting a drop of water in place)*, thus it will bring dreams to the one who wears it of places and times far beyond those of other mortals.

*She hands the jewel to the knight, who passes it through the candle flame.*

*Knight:* In the name of the sun king I bless and hallow this precious jewel. Within its heart I place a single flame taken from the sun's heart. *(He makes gesture of placing flame within.)* With this the jewel will bring courage to the heart of whoever shall wear it in honour, but to the one who is disloyal it will bring discovery and disgrace.

*He passes it across the altar to the warrior maid. She sprinkles it with salt.*

*Warrior maid:* With salt I grace this jewel drawn from the heart of the earth and within it I place a tear from the Eye of Shemataka. By this means the wearer will walk on the earth with her power and her authority, but should the wearer harm the earth, that same earth will cover their head until the world shall know them no more.

*She returns the jewel to the keeper.*

*Keeper:* I take this most precious thing into my keeping and it shall be given to that one who shall prove most worthy of it. It may not be taken by force, but may be given in love. It may not be coveted, but may be gazed on with joy. Taken by theft it will cause sorrow in the house of the thief. Used for evil it will turn upon the user and the land shall no longer hear their name.

*He encloses it within his hands and the priestess puts her hands over his. They speak together:*

Let the eye of the sun behold this consecration and stand witness. Let the eye of the moon behold this consecration and stand witness. Let the winds beyond the earth behold this conse-cration and stand witness. Let the ancient trees of earth behold this consecration and stand witness. This night, this hour, this work, this rite is done.

*The jewel is wrapped in silk and placed in a bag of chamois leather and tied securely. The priestess takes the chalice and pours into it a little wine to mix with the water and hands it to the keeper.*

*Priestess:* Take and drink and pledge thy power to this rite.

*The keeper drinks.*

*Keeper:* I do so pledge my power to this rite.

*He returns the chalice to the priestess who hands it on to the knight.*

*Priestess:* Take and drink and pledge thy power to this rite.

*The knight drinks.*

*Knight:* I do so pledge my power to this rite.

*He returns the chalice to the priestess who now hands it to the maid.*

*Priestess:* Take and drink and pledge thy power to this rite.

*The warrior maid drinks.*

*Warrior maid:* I do so pledge my power to this rite.

*She returns the chalice to the priestess who drinks from it also.*

*Priestess:* I also do pledge my power to this rite.

*Keeper:* Who will attempt the quest to seek this jewel?

*Warrior maid:* I will attempt the quest, and I challenge the knight.

*Knight:* I will attempt the quest, and I accept the challenge.

*Keeper:* So will the quest begin. Behave in all ways with honour and in love. If you should win, be loving in your victory. If you must lose, accept with grace and you will be blessed. Go in peace.

*The keeper takes the jewel and puts it away within his robe, then walks around the altar three times winding up the power, then declares the temple closed and the rite ended.*

The jewel remains in the hands of the keeper until the last day when he must hide it somewhere in the house, write down where he has hidden it and put this information in a sealed envelope in a drawer. When the outcome of the battle is known the winner may open the envelope, seek out their prize and wear it with pride.

# The Pathworking

Here in a cave is an ancient altar carved with many unknown symbols. On the altar stands a large copper bowl filled with flames, but no ordinary flames, they flicker with many colours – red, yellow, blue and green and a deep violet. The two before the altar are very conscious of themselves as a man and a woman of strength and determination, both trained as warriors, but with very different approaches to life and its mysteries. They have come here from two very different areas of this world to seek a magical jewel that is said to have great power. Each intends to gain that jewel but will have to go through many tests to find it and claim it.

Before them on the other side of the altar stands a man in a deep violet robe and a woman in green. Both are mature in appearance and with an aura of power about them. They are the keepers of the jewel, for only once in every thousand years may the jewel be won. On the death of its mortal owner it will return here to be held until the next claimant.

The flames die down, and lying within the bowl is a key. This will open the door to the first test. The knight and the warrior maid look at each other, wondering who will be given this key, but the keeper priest tells them that it must be shared, for the only way to the jewel is through co-operation. This is not exactly welcome news, but they agree. The woman takes the key and puts it in a leather pouch at her waist. They both kneel for the blessing of the keepers and bow their heads. For a moment they feel the light touch of hands, and then a little laugh. When they look up, they are alone, there is no altar, no fire, nothing but the cave lit by a single torch.

The man takes the torch and the two of them look around. There are many tunnels leading away from where they stand, but by which one did they enter? They were led here by the keepers but they have gone. Which tunnel is the right one? The knight looks for footprints but there are none. With a sigh of exasperation the woman grabs the torch from the man and sets off down the nearest tunnel. The man perforce must follow or be left in the dark. The two search for a long time and the torch is dying down when the man sees high above, set into the rock, a narrow ledge and a door.

He starts to climb, the woman following until suddenly the rock is smooth with no more hand or footholds. The ledge is still some nine or ten feet above them. The man motions the woman to his side and tells her to use him as a ladder. He will hold her weight until she can reach the ledge. She places her foot on his bent knee and springs lightly upward. With a knee to his shoulder she can just reach the ledge and place the now dim glow of the torch on it to guide her. It takes all her strength to haul herself up but she manages to do so and hurries to the door. The key fits and the door swings open. The man waits below – she can leave him here if she wishes and go on to the next sign that will lead to the jewel.

For a moment the instinct of self-preservation rules, then she returns to the ledge and lies flat, using her strong leather belt as a rope. The man grasps it and the struggle begins. He is much heavier and it taxes the woman's strength to hold him as he hauls himself up to the ledge. At last his hands grasp the top and for a moment he hangs free, then a last effort brings him up to safety. They rest for a moment and as they do so the torch flickers out.

The darkness is absolute and the man takes the woman's hand in his own. Together they feel their way towards the door. Progress is slow as they make their way along the new tunnel. It slopes upward however and they hope it will lead to the outside. As they walk they begin to hear a sound like a great roar, then as they get nearer they recognize it as the sound of rushing water. The tunnel ends abruptly and they find themselves standing on a small ledge beside an underground waterfall that enters a river below. However the river is flowing towards a cave mouth that lets in light and air. The only way out is down.

The woman wants to jump right away, but the man says, 'No, first we must take off our cloaks and wrap them tightly around our swords, otherwise the weight will drag us down. This way if we have to, we can let them go.'

Once ready they look at each other and the man holds out his hand. The woman shakes her head and leaps. The man follows.

The water is icy cold and swift-flowing and within minutes they are carried to the cave mouth and out into the air. The river flows through a gorge with high cliffs on either side and for a long time all their strength is used to keep afloat. Then the river widens and slows down and they come to the end of the gorge. There they struggle ashore and fling themselves down to rest. After a while the woman sits up and begins to scout around. It is getting dark and although she can see the marks of a path, it would be better if she started tomorrow at first light.

She looks around to see if there is anything to eat and finds some roots and berries which she eats. A sudden leap of flame attracts her attention. The man has gathered some wood and with a flint from his pouch has made a fire. The thought of warmth is enticing, so she hastily finishes her last few berries and walks back to the edge of the river. The two cloaks are hung over branches by the fire drying slowly, and the man's clothes are also hung there. In the now fading light she can see him standing in the river looking intently down at the water. In his hands he carries a sharpened stick. With a yell he stabs down and brings up a wriggling silver fish which he throws on to the shore.

The woman sits by the fire hugging herself to keep warm, and soon the man returns. Totally unselfconscious of his nudity, he threads four fish on a stick and positions them over the fire. He tells her to dry her clothes but she refuses to undress. He shrugs and goes to get more wood. He has noticed the berry juice around her mouth and is angry that she kept them all for herself when he was hungry too. However, he has the fish and intends to eat them all himself.

The smell of the food cooking is mouth-watering and the woman edges closer to the fire. The man slides a fish off the stick and tucks into it with relish. Licking his fingers he reaches for the second fish. The small sound of her stomach rumbling makes the woman shift uneasily. The berries were not very filling, but she would not ask for a fish if her life depended on it.

In a tower high on the mountain the two keepers watch in a silver scrying bowl and smile at each other. They breathe on the water and the image clouds over.

The man burps comfortably and reaches for the third fish, while the woman looks away. There is a touch on her arm and she looks round to see the fish laid neatly on a broad leaf being offered to her. She thinks of refusing, but her stomach protests and she takes the food and eats ravenously. The fourth fish is offered and accepted in silence and when she has finished the man leans over, gently removes the remains of a berry from her cheek and smiles.

The cloaks are dry enough to sleep in now and the two unwilling partners wrap themselves up and fall asleep. Before dawn they wake and, shivering in the cold wind, they begin to walk along the path the woman found last night. The way is hard and rocky and leads over scrubland and desolate moors. They rest at noon and then struggle on. The ground changes and becomes wet and boggy and without warning the man becomes trapped in a morass that slowly begins to suck him down. The woman looks round for a tree, a branch, anything that she can use to reach him, but there is nothing. He tries not to struggle but there is fear in his eyes. He tells her to go on and leave him, not wanting her to see his fear, but she will not. She remembers the warm fire, the fish, and the gentleness of the man. She stands up and draws her sword. The man looks up and nods, thinking that she has decided to kill him cleanly rather than let him die slowly in this stinking bog.

The woman reaches up and draws out the amber-headed pins that hold her hip-length hair in a tight knot. With a sweep of her sword she slices through the thick braid as close to her head as she can, then she stabs the sword deep into the firm ground she stands on and ties her belt to it. Holding on to this she edges out as far as she can and throws one end of the braid out to him. He grabs it and with renewed hope begins to pull himself from the grip of the morass.

Inch by inch they struggle to get him on to dry land until at last they both lie exhausted on safe ground. They fall asleep there, too tired to walk any more. The man wakes to the sound of weeping, and sees the woman sits holding her lovely braid in her hands with tears running down her face. Her hair had never before been cut, and was her pride and her joy. The man takes it from her and carefully wraps it into a coil and places it in his pouch. Then he lifts her muddied hands to his lips and kisses them. He owes her his life and she has sacrificed her pride for him.

Together they go on side by side. In the days that follow they go through many tests and face many dangers. Sometimes it is the woman's intuition that helps them find the path, sometimes it is the man's skills that are needed. They grow together in the knowledge of their friendship and begin to understand each other more and more. They take turns in hunting for food and gathering firewood. The woman teaches the man to wash clothes and weave leaves into a sleeping mat; he teaches her to read weather signs. They practise their swordplay together and learn much from each other's coaching. Once the man makes the woman a pair of sandals from the hide of a deer and leggings to protect her from the rocks and brambles. She has found out he has a sweet tooth, and when she finds a store of honey she gets badly stung trying to get it. Later they eat it together and he kisses her swollen face plastered with mud to cool the stings. One day he brings her a few small flowers, on another some dried berries he has clumsily strung together into a necklace. She carves him an amulet from a discarded antler and doses him with bitter herb bark when he eats the wrong kind of roots. Sometimes in the night, when he thinks she is asleep, he takes the braid of hair from his waist pouch and holds it to his face.

With each test they come nearer to the place of the jewel and one night by their fire they sit close together and talk about the quest. It is said that the jewel, besides giving power to the tribe that owns it, will give one wish to its holder. They talk about this until the fire dies down and it seems very natural to curl up in each other's arms to keep the last of the warmth. Sometime in the night the man wakes to find the woman cradling his head on her soft bare breast. She lies naked beside him and smiles at his sudden shyness as he tries to hide his arousal from her eyes. She is in her power as a woman and intends to lay claim to the man she has come to love as a friend and companion, as an equal and as a mate. Under the blessing of the full moon the warrior maid offers on equal terms the gift of herself, and the knight accepts and offers himself in turn to her.

They wake to find themselves in a castle high on a mountain. Fresh clothes and food are ready to hand. They descend into the great hall to find the keepers waiting there. Together they go to the chapel and there on the altar lies the magical jewel, a golden eye set in a ring of rubies. The pupil of the eye is a flawless emerald. The keepers ask who will take the jewel as they both have a claim to it. The two companions turn and face them. They do not want the jewel, for they have enough power in their combined strength and in their new-found love for each other. They will leave it here for others to win and go to seek their own life beyond the mountain. Their magical jewel is each other.

The keepers are not surprised at all and ask them to come to the altar. There they bless them and consecrate them for their lives ahead. To the knight who has learned not to despise a woman's strength of purpose and her courage they give a sword of mercy and to the woman who has learned to trust a man and to acknowledge his strength as a complement to her own they give a sword of justice. Then they pass over to them their own symbols of authority and tell them that now it is their turn to guard the magical jewel. Their love has set the keepers free and now they can go on to their own destiny.

Left in the chapel the lovers who were once opponents become the keepers. The jewel glows with fire. Its power reaches out to touch and enclose them and when it dies down the priestess's hair once more ripples past her waist. The keeper twines its shining length in his hands and draws her to him. Far away on the mountain road two people stop their horses and look up at the castle, then at each other and smile. They ride on towards their own future and leave the present behind.

# Ritual 7

# THE GRAIL OF GRACE

## The Programme

The next ritual is placed in Chesed on the Tree of Life, the sphere of the square and the number four, the sphere of organization, spiritual achievement, responsibility and maturity. It is the place of the Inner Plane Adepti, those teachers who willingly give up their right to a higher and finer level in order to teach humanity through contact on the astral and mental levels.

Here the man and the woman are approaching a much deeper area of their relationship. No longer are they content with just the physical and the emotional bonding, now there is a deeply felt need to seek out the masculine and feminine within themselves and to bond together in a four square relationship that will bring a spiritual strength to their physical and sexual bonding. At this point those who are undertaking these rituals should pause and ask themselves if their relationship, marriage or partnership is deep enough and true enough to go further. If you cannot be 100 per cent sure, then you are better not going further. There is no shame or failure in recognizing that a relationship may at some time in the future break up. I am not saying that unless you feel you are going to be together for 'eternity' you cannot work these rituals. What I *am* saying is, the rituals from now on will *bind you together for better or worse during this life*, and if any karmic debts are incurred you will be drawn back together very quickly to expiate them. You may divorce later or your partnership break up, but you will never be entirely free of each other, the bond will always be there. Therefore as your teacher and your temporary guardian through the medium of this book, I ask you to be sure.

Too many people regard sex as something casual to be indulged in and then forgotten. Nothing could be further from the truth. Every contact we make from the once only, 'Sorry, my fault,' when you bump into a stranger in the supermarket, to the commitment of the marriage bed, results in what is called an 'arc thread' linkage. An arc thread is an astral filament that attaches two people together. It can also attach people to things, pets, places, money, etc. The fleeting touch will soon thin out and fall away, but the deeper, repeated attachments can and do take a lifetime to break, if then.

The deepest contact two people can make is a sexual one. After all they are sharing their bodies with each other, and sharing the body fluids that flow through them, to say nothing of the astral, mental and spiritual fluids. The most fleeting of sexual contacts will result in a very strong arc thread and if by any chance the other person is aware of them and how they can be used, you are like a fish on a hook and you can be reeled in. If you are strong-willed you may be able to break them, if not, you will find yourself returning to that person again and again even if you do not wish to do so.

A man who habitually consorts with prostitutes or a woman who 'sleeps around' will quickly acquire the appearance of a fly tightly bound with spider's silk on the astral. The aura becomes unpleasantly sticky and friends and family begin to feel uncomfortable in their company. It can take a long time to get rid of such things – always providing you know how and are willing to spend the time and effort on doing it.

These rituals have not been written to titillate jaded appetites into new sexual fervour, they have been written to show that sex is neither degrading nor dirty when used in the right way, nor is its use incompatible with religious belief and practice. But if you intend to go further, please understand that the higher rituals will create a bond between you and make you more fully aware of your responsibilities to each other. The first and second rituals showed you how sex can be used in ritual, the third and fourth introduced you to the idea that sex has a much higher form, that its power can link people through time and space, and that it has a divine aspect. The fifth gave you your first glimpse of sex in its spiritual sense, a belonging so deep that it can transcend death. The sixth showed you that laughter, fantasy and fun also has a place and that fear of sex can be an illusion. Now you are attempting the seventh ritual of the series and seven has always been a magical number. This ritual is no exception. Here is a threshold: be careful how you cross it.

The Grail of Grace is in one way a coronation of The Empress and Emperor of the Major Arcana, at the same time it is the *hieros gamos*, the sacred marriage. The ritual is in two quite distinct parts. For the first part you will need two other people to work with you and when their part is done they should depart quietly, leaving the newly-made king and queen to work the second part. They

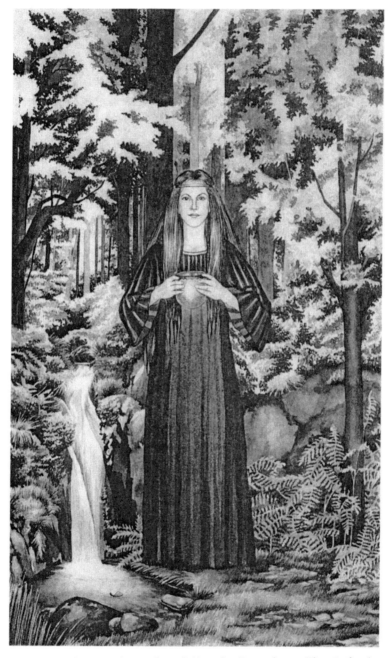

*Figure 18:* The Grail Maiden *(Miranda Gray,* from *The Arthurian Tarot)*

should be people who know enough to work well within a sacred location and who are trained enough not to make stupid remarks when their work is done and yours is just beginning.

You will need to prepare two rooms. Neither needs to be a 'temple' as such, but in both there must be enough room to move around. In the first room place a small square table for an altar with four chairs at the quarters, leaving room to walk right around the altar. This should be covered with a white cloth and then a smaller gold cloth. On this put a small vial of anointing oil and a golden ribbon long enough to bind two hands together in the east, a chalice of wine in the west, a small plate with two pieces of bread sprinkled with salt in the north, and a censer, incense and a candle in the south. In the centre place a lit altar lamp. Have two crowns to fit the heads of the king and queen ready to hand in the west. These can be made of card and gold foil with decoration as you wish, but make them to the very best of your ability.

In the bedroom place a bottle of wine and some food near the bed and scatter flower petals on the lower sheet. Fill the room with sweet smelling herbs and flowers and a carefully selected incense. The partners should buy two small pieces of jewellery for each other – medallions or rings to wear during magical work or anything that will give pleasure and be a reminder of the ritual. Needless to say, these should be kept as a surprise until the right time. Both partners should wear white robes and be naked beneath them. The priest and priestess should also be robed, but no specific colour is required.

With this ritual we return to the usual programme: no sexual contact between the partners and morning and evening exercises. The following is to be done by both partners: each day buy or pick a piece of fruit, a brightly-coloured vegetable or a sprig of herb for the next morning. On waking stretch every muscle as far as you can then relax, take away the pillow and roll your head gently to the right and to the left. Turn over and raise yourself on your hands and knees. Now arch the spine right up and push the head down so you are looking under your body, then put the head back and arch the spine the other way. Do this three or four times. Now you should be reasonably wide awake. Sit either on the floor on a folded blanket in the lotus position or, if it is more comfortable, on a straight-backed chair in the God form position. Place the fruit/vegetable in front of you.

Consider how you react to the world around you in five ways: by sight, smell, taste, sound and texture. This meditation point in front of you embodies all these things, yet how much do you know about them?

Close your eyes and see if you can recall clearly in your mind's eye the size and shape and colour of the object. If you think that is easy remember there are some people who cannot visualize at all. Can you remember where the shading comes without looking? Has it any flaws? Any discolouration? How big is it in relation to, say, your clenched hand? Now look and see how well you have visualized it. Give yourself marks out of ten.

Now try smell. Close your eyes again and try to recall the smell of that object. You can easily recall the smell of an apple or an orange, but what about a cabbage or a fresh carrot? What is the difference in smell between a sprig of marjoram and one of thyme? Try to bring the smell of your object to mind, then open your eyes, take it in your hand and sniff it. Try and impress that scent on your memory banks.

Touch is next. Again close your eyes and try to feel the texture of your object without touching it. The slightly slippery feel of a cabbage leaf is quite different from the roughness of a kiwi fruit. Again reach out with your mind and try to make that contact. Then open your eyes and hold it, and impress its texture in your mind. Always give yourself marks out of 10.

Now for sound. Did you think there was no noise to a carrot or an apple? Try rubbing your fingers along a carrot and hear the squeak, quite a different squeak from that of a turnip or an apple. Try opening your eyes and moving it from hand to hand and hear how the different shape and weight makes a different sound as it hits your hand.

The last sense of course is taste. Think of biting into the object and chewing it. Try to recall every detail of the taste. Is it sour, sweet, dry, bitter, sharp or bland? Is the taste different when you bite from when you chew? Does it have an after-taste? When you have thought about all this take a bite and really think about the taste in your mouth. You possess five miracles in your five senses yet half the time you do not even think about it.

The evening exercise is done together as a pair and is designed to bring about a greater awareness of your partner in a way similar to that of the morning session. Put down a soft blanket, and make sure the room is comfortably warm. You will also need some cushions or pillows. The exercise takes about 20 minutes in total.

Decide who will be first to observe. That person wears a robe or loose comfortable clothing. The other partner is nude and lies down on the blanket with a cushion or pillow under the head and one under the knees, lifting them slightly so that the knees are apart. The observer sits alongside them and at right angles. The one reclining must relax and close their eyes. The observer now begins to look at their partner, starting with the feet and gradually working their way up the body. Notice every little detail, from the smallest freckle to the lines on the throat and face. *Do not touch any part of the body at any time.*

You may bend over to see more closely so long as you do not touch. Continue this observation for 10 minutes in silence. Your task is see your partner as never before. Now change places and repeat the exercise.

It is of course expected that you will both behave with dignity during this exercise. You are offering your partner the gift of looking at your body with no distractions, simply looking and admiring and loving with your eyes. You might call it 'silent worship'.

On the second evening repeat the instructions, but this time lie down beside your partner and try to catch the scent of their bodies. A word here: of course you will want to bathe before this, but *do not apply any scent, use scented soap or talc or even a deodorant.* The real body scent is a potent aphrodisiac and must be allowed to come through. Change places after 10 minutes.

On the third evening ask your partner to read from a book and listen to their voice. Do not listen to the words, just to the cadences of the voice. Listen for traces of an accent or a phrase they use very often. Ask yourself what is the most personal or recognizable thing about their voice. After 10 minutes change over.

On the fourth evening we come to taste. I am not recommending cannibalism . . . but if you lick your partner's hand, face or body you will find that their skin has a very distinctive taste and that it will vary over the whole body. This however does not extend into oral sex: remember you are celibate for the rest of this week.

The fifth evening is for touch and this is placed last because of its obvious erotic potential. The passive partner should not move but allow the observer to touch as they please. Do not press hard or attempt to arouse your partner, just touch lightly but firmly as and where you wish. Learn the texture and surface of your partner. Try touching with your eyes closed and eyes open. Change over after 10 minutes.

The intention of this ritual is to bring about a complete recognition of each other as divine beings in potential. In many ways this ritual is similar to that of the third (Hod) but on a higher arc. You may be either married or living as partners in love, but this ritual will be a marriage on three levels: on the physical within a sacred circle, on the level of the anima and animus, and on the higher mental/spiritual level as beings who are potentially divine. Remember that at the end of the last ritual you became the keepers of the magical jewel. That jewel has another name – it is called Love.

# The Grail of Grace

## Sphere = Chesed. Keynote = Knowledge of One's Divine Self.

*When the temple is ready and prepared all gather at the altar. The high priest in the east and the high priestess in the west embody the anima and animus of the two undergoing their sacred nuptials. The man and woman are in the south and north. The altar light and the incense are lit. All face the east and bow.*

*High priest:* Within this place all is peace, all is light, all is love. We welcome the great archangels and elemental Malachim and invite them to share with us this sacred moment in time.

*He makes three circles around the temple and then proceeds to open the quarters using the pentagrams and the Qabalistic Cross. Then he turns to the altar and knocks two batteries of five.*

*High priest:* I declare this temple open and the intention of the rite is the sacred marriage blessed by the grail of grace. Man and woman come now to the east to be hallowed and made holy as was the custom in the ancient days when the priest kings were wed.

*The couple move to the east and take their place with their backs to the east and facing the high priest. They kneel down before him.*

*High priest:* Think well upon the intention of this ritual for it is a marriage beyond that of earthly law. Open yourselves to the great rays of love, wisdom and power that you may be lifted above the level of earth.

*Pause.*

Hold out your right hands.

*They do so and the high priest anoints them with oil.*

Hold out your left hands.

*They do so and these also are anointed.*

Lift up your heads that the mark of the seraphim may be placed upon your brows.

*The high priest draws the symbol of the winged serpent on each forehead. Now they stand.*

Upon your feet also shall you be marked, that your way may always be made safe before you.

*He marks the arches of their feet with oil.*

Woman, thou art made in the image of the Goddess, glorious and beautiful, strong and full of wisdom. In thy strength forget not those who have need of thee and who call thee 'priestess' and 'mother'. See thy complement in man as a companion and lover, for in love are you made whole as in the beginning. See in him your inner masculine self and rejoice. Man, thou art made in the image of the God. Uphold the ancient laws and protect those who have no strength of their own. Thou art upright and loyal, thou art defender and judge. Use the sword with mercy and the crook with justice. In this woman is thy life made complete as hers is made complete in thee. See in her your inner feminine self and rejoice. Let the sacred words of the east be spoken.

*The man and woman turn to each other and hold hands. They kiss.*

*Woman:* Thou art my inner self and in thee am I made whole. In the east I make my promise to thee of support and love, for here I am strong and clear-sighted. Like the sun at dawn I rise in glory to meet thee, body to body, heart to heart, mouth to mouth and soul to soul.

*Man:* Thou art my inner self and in thee am I made whole. In the east I make my promise to thee of strength and protection, for here I am gentle and wise. Like the sun at dawn I rise in glory to meet thee, body to body, heart to heart, mouth to mouth, and soul to soul.

*The high priest turns to face the west and bows.*

*High priest:* Priestess of the grail, into thy hands I place this man and woman, hallowed by the east and made ready for thee. By thy power invoke the grail of grace.

*The high priestess lifts the chalice and bows to the east, then turns to the west and holds up the chalice.*

*High priestess:* I invoke Nuit, Goddess of the starry void, Nuit of the fruitful womb and gentle hands. Look on this chalice, for it is humanity's symbol of thee and thy power. In thee are all women maintained in spiritual grace and all men made Gods. Thy chalice is the sacred space wherein man comes to meet his feminine self, where he may draw on wisdom and grace. Here he is conceived and formed, nurtured and secured against harm, from here is he expelled into the world, to here he may return to give homage and offer up his life force for thy use, if a woman will but grant him leave to enter her sacred space. Nuit, daughter, sister, wife, mother and Goddess, fill this chalice with thyself that those who drink may be filled with the inner and higher knowledge of the Tree of Life.

*She turns and calls the man and woman to the west.*

Come to me that I may bless and hallow thee.

*The high priest escorts them to the west where they stand with their backs to that quarter, facing the altar. The high priestess turns to face them, while the high priest stands behind them.*

*High priestess:* This is the grail of grace, filled with the power and passion of Nuit the eternal mother. In this you will pledge to reflect each other's inner self with truth, grace and gentleness. In taking this wine into yourselves you take also the great duality of male and female principles, for as the chalice is the mother of form, so the father is the wine that needs formation to manifest. Drink and be blessed, for in you the first parents have come full circle.

*The high priestess extends the chalice to the woman, who drinks deeply. Then, still holding the chalice, she speaks:*

Woman: I am woman, blessed and filled with grace. Within my body I hold the archetypal temple of life. In love and with the knowledge of our equality I make thee priest of that temple wherein the worship of the great duality may take place.

*She returns the chalice to the high priestess who lifts it up for a moment and then gives it to the man. He drinks, leaving about half a normal wine glass in it, then, holding it, he speaks:*

Man: I am man, blessed and filled with grace. My phallus is the key to the temple of life. In love and with the knowledge of our equality I accept the priesthood and the guardianship of that temple. On its altar I will offer myself and the life force within me.

*He returns the chalice to the high priestess. They rise and the high priest takes them back to their first places, leaving the woman in the north and taking the man to the south, then returning to the east.*

Woman: I am the earth, sweet and fertile. I offer thee bread and salt in token of our joining.

*She holds the plate of bread/salt over the altar. The man takes a piece and eats. The woman also eats a piece then returns the plate to the altar.*

Man: I am the sun at noon. I offer thee this sweet incense in token of our joining.

*He offers the censer over the altar and with his hand waves the smoke in her direction, then replaces it on the altar.*

*The high priest beckons them to come before him as before with their backs to the east. He then lightly binds their two left hands together with the ribbon. The high priestess brings the chalice and gives it to the woman in her free hand. The high priest lights the candle from the altar light and gives it to the man in his free hand. The high priestess also brings the two crowns and she and the high priest place them on the heads of the man and woman, making them The Emperor and Empress.*

High priestess: Let earth and heaven rejoice, for the two shall become one, the key shall open the door of the ancient temple, and the temple will once more know the fire of worship upon its altar.

*The Empress raises the chalice and holds it out to The Emperor. He holds the candle above it.*

High priestess: Let all the holy ones stand witness to this sacred joining. That which was broken in two shall become whole. The temple shall hear the voice of its priestess raised in joy. Blessed be this night and those who share it.

*The Emperor upends the candle and slowly brings it down into the chalice until it is doused in the wine.*

*Emperor:* I, man, take thee, woman, as my love and equal.

*Empress:* I, woman, take thee, man, as my love and equal.

*High priest:* As the candle is to the male . . .

*High priestess:* So the chalice is to the female . . .

*All:* And the one into the other shall give blessing and life. Selah.

*They all return to their places. The ribbon is loosed. The high priest performs the closing ritual and retraces the three circumambulations winding up the power, then stands before the altar and gives the knocks in two batteries of five.*

*High priestess:* The rite is done. Let us depart in peace.

*The high priest and priestess depart, leaving The Emperor and Empress together for a few minutes. The others leave the house and the rite then continues.*

*Emperor:* The grace of the chalice is upon us. Will you grant me entrance to the temple?

*Empress:* In the grace of the chalice we will trust. I will grant you entrance to the temple.

*They leave the temple and return to their prepared chamber. There they may have something to eat and to drink, but not too much. They lay the crowns and their robes aside, then lie side by side and recall the evening exercises. However this time they are used for the purpose of arousal and the five senses are brought together and lifted into the higher levels. During the love play the 'litany' is used as the sense of hearing, oils as the sense of smell, wine as the sense of taste, caresses as the sense of touch and the use of visualization of each other as The Emperor and Empress of the Tarot as the sense of sight.*

*Emperor:* In thee am I made complete and whole. Thou art a sweet fountain of water in the desert, thou art the grass that yields the power of the earth, thou art the dawn of light upon the mountains of the moon and the song of the phoenix as she rises from the flames. With thee all things are possible. Open the doors of the temple that I may worship and offer my sacrifice of love.

*Empress:* Without thee I am alone and lost. Thou art the vine-bearing grapes that quench my thirst, thou art the tree that shades me from the noon sun, thou art the guardian at the door of my sacred place. Take thou the key of life and approach the temple, there will I meet thee and worship with thee.

*When the temple that is the body of the woman is well prepared, the key that is the phallus enters the lock that is the vagina and The Emperor proceeds to the adytum within the temple. Approach the joining with the thought held in mind of the sanctity of the act, the hallowing of the sacred marriage that has gone before, and also the thought that your inner male and female selves will share in this moment. Let your emotions lift you from the physical to the astral and perceive the angelic forms that surround you. When the astral level has been established, lift again to the mental where the brilliant forms of the Four Holy Living Creatures become visible at the quarters. Pause at each shift in the levels, then proceed again. Wait now until the force of the sexual climax is almost upon you, and at that precise moment allow its power to lift you one last time to the spiritual level. Let your minds, hearts and bodies enter the light on the wings of your sexual power – not only the bodies but also the inner selves will join at this moment. It is the marriage of the anima and the animus as well as your own marriage. Fix your attention on the starry figure of Nuit as her body curves over the horizon. The transmutation of male and female into God and Goddess is, for a brief moment, made fully manifest. Then allow yourselves to glide gently down the levels and rest in each other's arms, secure and without fear.*

# The Pathworking

It is night. We stand near the top of a mountain. Behind us rises a temple of white stone crowned with a cupola. The perfume of incense drifts through the open doors and we can see the gleam of candles lighting the interior. The rise and fall of voices can be heard chanting an ancient hymn of praise. The temple is being prepared for a special ceremony.

Far below us the chant is echoed by many voices and we see two lines of moving figures, one in white robes and the other in blue. They come from opposite sides of the valley where two large buildings stand, alike in size and shape. The one on our right flies a banner bearing the device of a silver grail on a blue background, the one on our left has a banner showing a flaming torch on a white background.

The two lines approach the winding road leading up the mountain to the temple and merge into a double line of blue and white robed figures. Their voices blend in subtle harmony, the baritones and basses of the men lightened by the tenor range, while the altos and sopranos of the women add an otherworldliness to the minor key of the music.

Each person carries a torch to light their way and as they approach we see those in white robes are men and those in blue are women. A voice behind us bids us welcome and we turn to see a man in a golden robe, his shaven head gleaming in the light streaming from the open door of the temple. At his side stands a woman, her blue robes embroidered with tiny silver stars, her long dark hair braided about her head. They stand with us looking down at the approaching line and explain that tonight The Emperor and The Empress will be crowned and wed, and that they have been chosen from the two temples in the hidden valley to fulfil this task. It has been so from time immemorial, since the last Atlantean temple disappeared beneath the cold waves.

The first of the singers reaches the top of the path and walks towards the door over the stone pathway smoothed over the centuries by the tread of countless feet. The singers' faces are joyful and serene, their eyes full of hope.

At the door helpers have set up two large stone jars of water and as each pair approaches the temple they take the torches and douse them in the charged water. We wait until all have entered the temple, then enter with the high priest and high priestess.

Within we are dazzled by the light: the whole temple is lit by hundreds, maybe thousands of candles and the air is heavy with incense. The altar is formed of two cubes, one on top of the other. The lower cube is white marble, the top its counterpart in black. Cut into the marble on every side are golden letters in a strange script. We are escorted to the front of the gathering and as we pass the people bow in a wave of motion like a ripple on a quiet sea.

At each side stands a golden screen and from behind them come two processions. There is a sudden silence and we see in the middle of each procession a figure dressed in simple white robes of almost transparent linen. These two figures are a man and a woman, she with her hair flowing loose and unbound, he clean shaven, his dark hair bound with a silver filet. At the altar the two approach the high priesthood and the ceremony begins.

Each in turn, the chosen ones are stripped and washed with holy water in which sea salt has been dissolved. Then they are anointed and hallowed with oil as were the priest-kings of Atlantis when they wed the chosen priestesses of the Naradek temple. We understand now that we are present at the nuptials of the sun and moon.

Crowns of gold, heavy with gems, are set upon their heads. The head of the young Empress bows for a moment under the weight, but we see her companion lift her hand to his lips and she straightens up and smiles at him. Hers will be the greater burden, for she will become the archetypal priestess and mother of the world. The Emperor will rely on her judgement and her intuition to guide him in his work.

They turn to face the congregation and the sword and sceptre are placed into the hands of The Emperor, and the orb and shield into the hands of The Empress. From here they are taken to the two thrones set at the very top of the temple.

Now a great silence comes upon us. The doors open and we feel a strange pressure clutch our hearts. Down the aisle comes a procession of beings. They shine like suns, gleam like stars, their faces are the faces of angels, for that is what they are. Two by two they approach the throne and make their obeisance to the two who will rule the earth for this aeon. After them come the stately Malachim, the kings of the elements and their subjects, followed by the archangels whose faces are so bright we must look away. Then the Gods and Goddesses, to us creatures of myth and legend, but here beings of substance and glory. Last of all one presence comes, before whom all, even the newly-made royalty bows. Metatron, the mighty Angel of the Throne, Keeper of the Name Unspoken, comes to bless the young pair and to make them not only royal but man and wife.

The archangel takes their hands and binds them together with the cord from about its waist. With hands that glow like fire it blesses them. In words that hang like tiny flames above the altar it pronounces them man and wife before the eternal duality. It takes up the great chalice, breathes upon the wine and gives it them to drink. This is the final sacrifice, for with this sip of wine their mortality will be gone and for this aeon they will live on and on past the ending of those they love until two more shall come to take their place. They will have great need of each other, for soon all they know and love will be gone. Theirs is a heavy burden.

Metatron turns to those gathered and lifts the chalice in blessing. For a brief moment the being's eyes, lambent, glowing, awesome, touch ours and we are caught in their power. The light streams from them and blinds us, growing brighter and brighter until we lose consciousness and slip into a blessed darkness that is soft and warm.

Slowly we return to ourselves. Around us are familiar things, our own things, our own surroundings. We are back on our own level of existence, but knowing we will be forever changed by what we have seen.

# Ritual 8

# THE RITE OF CRYSTAL

## The Programme

Life, this sphere, is indicated by a circle of dotted lines. Da'ath is not really there, but where it *is*, or might be, has been debated since the Western Tradition began to use the Qabalah in its practices. It has been claimed that Da'ath is the Tiphereth of a Tree in another dimension, or that it represents either the 'fallen' earth sphere of Malkuth or the lower arc of Yesod. There are variations in almost every book on the subject. I have decided to include it as a sphere of ritual because I have found it to be a place where paths from many levels and dimensions meet and cross and therefore it holds great power.

It also seemed fitting that the last four spheres should correspond to the elemental quarters in their many aspects. After much thought I saw that I would inevitably have to follow the lead of Binah as the sphere of water. Chocmah has always been considered a sphere of fire. This makes Kether, named as the point of manifestation, also the element of air, and Da'ath becomes the perfected element of earth. The question was, what aspect of earth would best symbolize the ethereal Da'ath? The answer was the most beautiful of earth's gifts to humanity: the crystal.

All four of these rituals have a crystal as a central symbol. Da'ath, as the element of earth, will concentrate on the perfect union of the male/female polarities, while Binah as the form element of water will be the chalice-bearing feminine principle. Chocmah, the sphere of fire, will be male-orientated, dealing with the rod of power, the ithyphallic image of the Horned God. Kether, the last sphere, will use the vibrant air element, the Word of Creation from which all things emerge.

As can be seen from Fig 19, the Tree of Ecstasy is divided into three natural sections. Malkuth, Yesod, Hod and Netzach, the first four spheres and their rituals, form the image of a cup and may be

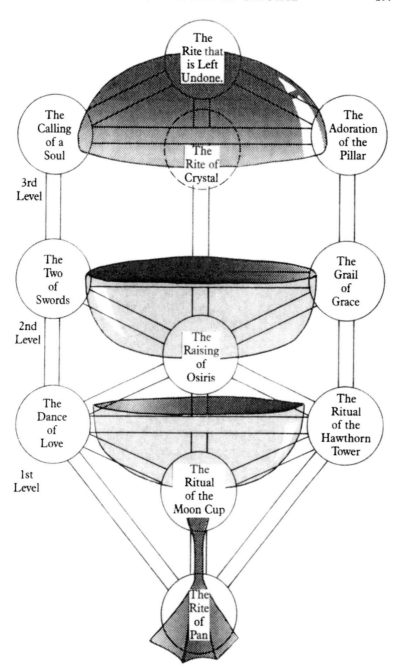

*Figure 19:* The levels of the Tree of Ecstasy

considered the first level of sexual magic. Here a period of adjustment to the idea of sex as a means of worship takes place before the next level is attempted. Tiphereth, Geburah and Chesed form the second level where the sexual power enters the higher astral and lower mental spheres. Here the bond that goes beyond the seen into the unseen and the unknowable becomes manifested. Here the idea of fantasy as a stepping stone to the mental spheres is offered to the mind as training aid. The Chesedic sphere and the symbol of the grail mark the end of the second level.

Da'ath can be regarded as a separate level, a borderline between what is known and what is yet to be experienced. However, it is best thought of as part of the third and final level where sexual magic becomes sexual mysticism and moves into the realm of pure creation. The intention of the Da'ath ritual is to bond the sexual partners with one of the oldest parts of their mother earth, the crystal world. It is also intended to make the crystals used in the rite the focus of an ongoing communication between the man and the woman and the world of the supernal triad.

Crystals, unlike rocks, actually 'grow'. They have a preordained structure according to type and grow slowly and carefully over great spaces of time. This makes them a very special part of nature. Despite their appearance, they are fragile and are easily damaged especially by rapid changes of temperature. They have been used by mankind for thousands of years and not only as gems for their beauty of shape and colour. They have the ability to hold and amplify vibrations from the human mind and other dimensions and have been used in the field of communications since the first 'crystal sets'. My father used to make them when he was still a schoolboy and well remembers the thrill of listening to the voices brought to him by the power of the little crystal.

There are many books available that will give you all the information you need on the use of crystals. The ones I use most frequently are *Crystal Healing: The Next Step* by Phyllis Galde (Llewellyn, 1989) and *The Crystal Workbook* by Ursula Markham (The Aquarian Press, 1988). The first mentioned is a small paperback that manages to pack a wealth of information into its pages and I recommend it highly.

For this ritual you will need two pieces of clear rock crystal, two pieces of blue lace agate, one piece of moonstone (for the woman) and a piece of either smoky quartz or snowflake obsidian (for the man) and one piece of rose quartz. The rock crystal will be used to amplify the forces around you during the ritual and make them visible to your psychic sight. The blue lace agate will give you inner peace and calm as you approach the spiritual levels of the work. The moonstone will help the woman to stay in touch with her femininity and her intuitional priestess self which is most important (remember The Lovers of the Tarot). 'The smoky quartz,' says Phyllis Galde, 'will initiate the basic primal forces of your body allowing you to better express your physical self.' Of the snowflake obsidian she says, '. . . it is said to sharpen both the internal and external vision and is one of the most important teachings stones of the New Age. It is the Warrior of Truth...' This is a good description of what the male partner will become through these rituals.

All the stones should be as perfect as possible and quite small – certainly no bigger than a fingernail at most. The moonstone, being more expensive, may be even smaller. The rose quartz should be a little larger and if possible polished into a smooth pebble shape. 'It is the gemstone of the heart chakra and important for the giving and receiving of love' – here again I quote from Phyllis Galde. Such a power makes it the ideal centrepiece for the ritual.

Instead of a God form or an angelic being you will be working this time with the Devas of the crystals. A Deva is a being of the angelic type usually appointed as an overseer or guardian of a place or an object of great beauty or veneration. This can apply to things like menhirs, stone circles, woods and forests, mountain ranges and gemstones.

The stones used in this ritual will become not only charged with the power of the rite, they will home in on the spiritual energy and the emotion that passes between you as a sexually polarized partnership. There will never be anything like them again, as they will be tuned into the pair bond built between you, which will be taken to even greater heights from now on. When you completed the Geburic fantasy ritual I *did* warn you that ahead lay a total commitment to each other for this life. You have already experienced a spiritual marriage and coronation, you have already gone through the physical and astral levels of sex and touched lightly on the lower mental, now you approach the spiritual levels and your dealings with that level must be truthful and sincere. You are entering the dimension that links physical sex to the power that creates stars and galaxies, and you *must* understand fully what you are getting into. Only complete honesty with each other and the forces with which you are now dealing will suffice.

I have asked a great deal of you during your progress through this book: I am now going to ask even more of you. This ritual will in effect take a full month to accomplish, though the ritual *itself* requires only an hour or so, and I am asking you to remain celibate throughout that month, starting on the first day of a new moon and finishing with the performing of the ritual on the first day of the next new moon. It is important that your sexual strength and emotional tension is built up as high as possible. If you feel you cannot do this, put the book aside until you have reached a point in your spiritual progress where you can do it. Remember there are three more rituals to accomplish that are going to test your strength even further. It is up to you to decide.

The exercises are almost the same for both partners and are divided into four lots of seven days starting with the first day of a new moon. Keep the crystals with you at all times and as close to your skin as possible. All except the rose quartz should be kept in a small cloth bag hung around your neck during the day and placed under the pillow at night.

Each morning of the first week take your crystals from under your pillow and take off any nightclothes you may be wearing. Take away the pillow, lie flat on your back and arrange the crystals along your body. The rock crystal goes between the eyebrows, the lace agate over the heart centre, the moonstone is placed directly over the womb and the smoky quartz or obsidian is placed between the penis and the scrotum. If the man experiences a morning erection then place the crystal on the scrotum itself and hold it there. We begin with the rock crystal.

With eyes closed concentrate on the feel of the crystal between your eyebrows. Feel its coolness growing warm. Now imagine that it is putting out tiny crystal feelers that sink down into your head, seeking out the root of your inner sight. Let it grow slowly; you have a whole week for it to reach its goal. Feel the awareness of the crystal as it becomes part of you and learns to trust you. Let it move at its own pace for a short while and then ask it to stop and let it know that you will continue with this 'getting to know you' phase tomorrow. Now turn your attention to the agate. Follow the same pattern, allowing the crystal to send its tiny filaments down towards your heart centre gently and slowly. Remember that very few people will allow a crystal into their psycho-physical space, and this is a blessing beyond anything their tiny spirits could hope for. Now call a halt and again let the crystal know that it may continue its inward journey tomorrow.

The moonstone placed over the womb will grow down towards the centre of the feminine self. When your period occurs during this month feed the moonstone with a little of your menstrual blood, just gently rubbing it in with your fingertip. There is nothing distasteful about this fluid: it is part of you, part of your body and contains a great deal of your feminine power. Do not think of it as being dirty or unclean – by now both partners should be able to cope with their own and each other's body fluids without distaste. The moonstone will gradually make contact not only with the womb but with the vagina and the clitoris, in fact the whole of your sexuality will be attuned to the power of this stone. If you are male let your particular crystal send its roots inward to the perineum, a most important part of the body, especially in the male, and sometimes referred to as the Gate of Life and Death. Now gently remove the crystals and replace them in their bag. Allow the crystals to progress a little further each day for the first week.

During the second week the crystals, which will by now have made their full contact with the pineal, heart, and womb/genitals/ perineum centres, should be encouraged to communicate with you. In the same way that elementals are in contact with their elemental king and the regent or archangel of their element, so crystals are in contact with their Deva. Once the spirit of the crystal has made full contact with the visionary, emotional and creative centres they will begin to communicate with you through increased activity in the centres themselves and by responding to your mind touch each morning. Each and every crystal has a unique vibration similar to a personal name in our human species, and in time, if the full contact has been made, this will be revealed to you.

When crystals put down their tiny roots they leave a substance similar to a fine sand in the chakra, like a fingerprint or a signature. The parent stone may be elsewhere but you will always be in contact through the root substance left in the chakra. In this way you are always in touch with the Earth Mother for like the crystal in the old fashioned wireless, this crystal sand acts as an antenna. In people who are highly psychic the pituitary gland also holds a similar substance.

During the third week your task is to activate the crystal sand in each centre and use the crystal itself to focus the generated power outward. First try with the pineal. Focus from the centre and through the crystal towards a plant, a tree or a local beauty spot you know well. Use the power to show you the Deva of that plant, tree or place. Look carefully and try to impress it on your memory, then slowly close down. Now open the heart centre and focus through the agate. Reach out to the Deva and communicate with it. If you have need of it, ask for healing and strength and feel the power flow out to you. After a few minutes close the centre down. Now activate the last crystal, summon the creative power from within and focus through the stone. Ask the Deva to show you the inner working of the plant, tree or the place of its being. It may show you how it can be helped if it is in an area that is threatened. Now close down, but always check and make sure you have closed right down or you will get problems during the day.

During the last week place all three stones on the forehead and focus the inner visionary power through all of them. You will find, according to your strength, that you will be able to envisage a triune being composed of all three colours. These are the Devas of each crystal *type* combining their strengths. With practice you should be able to communicate with these beings and at a later date focus their powers and use them for many purposes: empathic healing of all kinds, seership and intuitive clairvoyance, and enhanced creative ability in your work and private life. Each day try to make your contact a little deeper and stronger.

Now for the rose quartz. This stone is the focus of the evening exercise to be done as a pair. Sit side by side in the God form position and hold the rose crystal in your linked hands. Concentrate on the crystal for a few minutes to let it know it is the focus of your thoughts. It may take a little time but you should soon begin to feel a response in the form of tiny images flickering at the edge of your inner vision. Let it continue and keep on sending quiet gentle thoughts along the lines of an introduction to a new friend. Do this for about 10 to 15 minutes then close down. Continue this through the first week until the crystal sends out a recognition image as soon as you begin.

During the second week ask the crystal to give you a picture of the rose quartz Deva and each day gradually build up the image until it is quite clear. To make sure you are working as a team, take turns in describing what you are seeing. Once the being is quite clear to your inner sight, use the inner focal points you have been given by the other crystals to communicate with it. Beings such as these have many lovely stories to tell and information to give about their crystal children.

The third week is spent communicating with the Deva about the ritual and the part it will play in that ritual. The rose quartz stone you are using each evening will be magnetized and attuned to the vibration of human love that reaches through the physical, astral, mental and spiritual levels. This is achieved by focusing the powers of the inner crystals on the rose quartz and consciously empowering it with insight and communication abilities, empathy and love, and creativity. This will raise its powers far beyond what is normal and enable it to do the work for which it is destined.

Each night during the last week put the rose crystal in your bed. Just place it in the middle and let it wander around while you sleep. When you sleep you will relax and your thoughts and energies will fill the crystal with your feelings, emotions and dreams. Each morning find the crystal and take it in turns to carry it with you through the day.

For the ritual itself you will need 12 rose-coloured candles and 12 more crystals of any kind. Maybe you already have some, but do not use them unless you are willing to give them up when the ritual is finished. For incense I would suggest 'Deva', specially made for this ritual by Golden Lotus Products.

# The Rite of Crystal

## Sphere = Da'ath. Keynote = Knowledge of One's Divinity.

*Prepare your bedroom with great care. If possible use a rose-coloured sheet, and if you have any large crystals place them around the room and put a candle by each one so it catches the light and reflects it around the room. Put the other candles in twos and threes to fill the room with soft shadows. If you have them, bring in some large mirrors and place them so that they will reflect the room, bed, candles and crystals.*

*Eat lightly and then prepare your ritual bath, adding a few drops of the appropriate oil to water that is nicely warm but not hot. Take one or two of the crystals into the bath with you and hold them. Lave them with the water and see how they glitter. Have you ever thought about their birth? Deep in the warm earth in the silence of millions of years they lie dreaming, then suddenly they are taken out into the light and exposed to the coldness of human life. A few, a very few, escape back to their birthplace, and even fewer are replaced with tender care, having been filled with grace and blessed. That is one of the intentions of this ritual.*

*When you have bathed and are ready to begin the ritual take the crystals you have carried with you for so long and place them on the pillows. Now take the other crystals and place them in groups at the four corners of the bed. Secure them lightly with clear tape if needed. Bind your rock crystals to your forehead with a ribbon or scarf, secure the agate over the heart with tape, and place the third stone in the hollow of the navel. So long as they have no very sharp edges they will not cut you.*

*Sit opposite each other with the rose quartz crystal by your side, the man cross-legged, the woman sitting with her knees apart and leaning back on her hands, her head thrown back. The man looks at her and, using his imagination, begins to arouse his male power. The woman moves from one position to another, enticing and inviting, offering herself to his eyes. Now he moves to her and begins to arouse her in turn, touching her face and the soft skin where the neck joins the shoulder and behind the ears. The inside of the arm, the inner thigh and the back of the knee are all packed with nerve centres and very sensitive. The woman in her turn caresses the man, paying particular attention to the place where the exposed glans is attached to the frenum, where the skin is held to the top of the glans itself. This is extremely delicate and needs to be touched carefully, but it is also sexually very sensitive. The scrotum and the point between the root of the scrotum and the anus are also highly erotic nerve points. Go slowly, and if you feel too aroused simply sit and look at each other until you can begin again. The raw sexual power you are giving out is being attracted by the crystals to themselves and stored as pure energy. Those crystals that are attached to your body are also soaking in this power.*

*The woman picks up the rose quartz crystal and passes it over her partner's body, covering it with the sexual sweat he has generated and collecting the tiny drop of moisture at the opening of the penis. Then the man takes it and does the same for the woman, placing it carefully in the tiny cavity of the clitoris to collect her sexual lubricants.*

*Then it is placed for the moment on the bed beside them and the man resumes his cross-legged position. The woman raises herself over him and slowly lowers her body until she can feel the tip of his penis at the entrance to her body.*

*Woman:* I am the gate of sweet delights. Behind me there is the corridor of joy leading to the hall of sacrifice. Enter the gate and be welcome.

*Man:* I am the key to the gate. I seek the pearl hidden from the eyes of man. Lead me onwards.

*The woman lowers herself again.*

*Woman:* Enter the corridor of joy and I will hold thee captive and call thee 'beloved'.

*Man:* Thou art the pearl I seek. I will hold thee and be held by thee in silken chains.

*Woman:* I have opened the hall of sacrifice. Leave the offering of your life force at my altar.

*Man:* To thee, image of the Great Mother, I offer sacrifice.

*The woman lowers herself completely onto the man's penis and fits her legs around his waist. Now they remain still, the woman using only her internal muscles to caress the male erection. They both begin to build up the Devas of the crystals until they can see them clearly with the inner sight. These beings then connect with the crystals set at the corners of the bed and build up a crystalline sphere that wraps the lovers around with a delicate inner level web of power. Once this is perceived they begin to build the Deva of the rose quartz, seeing it as growing taller and glowing with rose light. At this point the man takes the rose crystal and places it as close as possible to the point of joining.*

*Now the mating moves to its climax, but both partners must try to keep the Deva within their inner sight – not an easy task. As the sexual ecstasy approaches the Deva will glow brighter and brighter as the energy fills it.*

*As the lovers reach their moment of orgasm, they let their inner selves flow towards the Deva and join with it. The others also join them and human and crystal become one on the inner levels. At such a moment the matter that composes the two quite different species becomes one, just as it was before the universe exploded untold millions of years ago. Then it was just one immense mass of proto-matter, now for a fleeting second a few tiny particles of that mass come together once more. The crystals are filled with your creative energy and, more important, with your consciousness of the moment.*

*Allow yourselves to descend gently from the peak and rest a moment with the man's head on his partner's breast before withdrawal from her body. The Devas will slowly withdraw at the same time. They will be as sated as you, though not in the same way. You have offered them something they could never have hoped for, a moment's union with humanity. They are blessed by this to an extent we cannot fully understand. Place the crystals you are wearing under your pillow and leave the ones set at the corners for the night. The rose quartz should be placed between your pillows to act as a guardian.*

*The three personal stones you will keep with you until they tell you it is time for them to go, while the others should be gathered together and, with the rose quartz as their 'leader', taken to a place of beauty and if possible, remoteness. There they must be buried as deeply as possible. They will sink down into the earth, filled with your human sexual energy lovingly offered, and that energy will act as a communication beacon between the Earth Mother and her sister planets, and also between her and other human beings, if they are sensitive enough to hear her. Of course they will also be responsive to you if you visit this place again, for your energy pattern has become bonded to their crystalline consciousness and they will always be aware of you. Wherever you are on this planet, the crystals you blessed with your love will respond to your thoughts.*

*If you travel abroad often to different places, you might like to take crystals with you or buy them in that location and work the ritual again. By this means you can leave a cache of human-energy sensitized crystals wherever you go. In this way you can increase the earth's awareness and her ability to communicate with all other life-forms on this planet, and maybe even farther into the solar system.*

# The Pathworking

In your mind's eye build a doorway of shimmering emerald-coloured crystal. Set into the middle of this door is the golden symbol of an eye. At the moment it is closed, but as you approach it the eye opens to reveal a pupil of sapphire centred with an iris of onyx. The eye looks at you for a long moment as if judging your credentials, then it closes again and the door swings open.

Beyond you can see nothing but a grey mist shot through with many colours, but you can hear a sound that fills you with wonder. Imagine a thousand tiny silver bells, each one carefully tuned to a different note through all the major and minor keys. You can hear them far above and below your normal range of hearing.

You walk forward into the mist and the door closes silently behind you. You walk on and gradually the mist clears away and you find yourself on a wide grassy plain – at least you assume it is grass, certainly it is similar to grass, only it ranges in colour from deep purple to light lavender. Here and there you see tall plants that look rather like trees, but with feathers instead of leaves. Above you two suns circle in the sky, one a deep hot purple and the other much lighter. You walk towards the trees, intending to sit in the shade out of the bright light of the double sun. As you pass into the shade you see that the ground is covered with hundreds of crystals. Their colours range, like the suns, from dark purple amethyst to the palest of lavender pinks. They differ in size also and in shape, some being double, others single, yet others in groups of multiples.

You go to pick one up, but it starts to glow and flash through a range of shades of its basic colour. The air is filled with tiny bell-like sounds but, unlike those you heard earlier, these are discordant. Because you are on a higher level of being you are more aware of the finer senses, and you realize that these are sounds of distress and even fear. You withdraw your hand and instead sit quietly beside the largest of the crystals. Leaning against a tree, you calm your mind into a state of meditation.

At first the sounds seem to have no form or meaning but gradually you begin to distinguish their pattern. You make an effort to reach a level where you can understand and with a sudden clarity it all falls into place. The largest crystal is speaking to you. It asks about you, what kind of life form you are, where you come from, how it feels to be able to move from place to place of your own accord. It asks if you mean its fellows harm.

You answer as best you can, explaining your form, your planet, for by now you realize you are not on Earth. You try to describe your life and work, then ask the crystals to explain their ways. There is a short silence then the large crystal asks you to pick it up and hold it to your forehead. For a moment you experience a sharp pain in the deepest part of your brain, then suddenly you can hear the thoughts of the crystals much more clearly and see images.

They show you their world and you see that there are many places like this but that the crystals are of different colours, just as on Earth we have people of different colour. You learn that they have a much longer day than ours, almost five times as long, and that the suns act as a stimulus for them mentally. For them a day in the sunlight means growth both in size and knowledge.

Their knowledge is of a different kind to ours, more aligned to what we would call philosophy. They have no handicrafts as we have, but they are artists who reflect light from within themselves and use it to create a harmony of light and sound, much as a symphony would be for us. They also have great 'thinkers' who probe the universe around their planet and in their thoughts link with other life forms. The crystals ask politely if you would mind allowing one of their 'thinkers' to join its thoughts with yours. Think about this: they will then know everything about you and your world. Are you proud of it and what your life form has done to that world? How will these crystal life forms react to the knowledge that on Earth we wear their kind as ornaments?

The crystals wait silently, then one of the smaller ones sends you a thought: 'We understand. You are sending thoughts of distress, you think we may not like what we will find. That is true, but we have learned that within the universe there are many things we do not like or understand; however, if the One has ordained these things it is because they are needed to bring some change into the universe. We will not judge, we only wish to know, and, if possible, to understand.'

So you open your heart and mind to the crystals and your brain is filled with light. A myriad different pieces of knowledge enter and leave your mind. You realize that the communication is two-way, that you can now understand much more about them. After a while the interaction is withdrawn and all is silent.

Much later the larger crystals make contact again and you find that they are very flattered that we use the powers of their form in our communication work. They are not too happy about the idea of jewellery but they like very much the fact that the diamond is a gift of love. They ask about the human way of love and reproduction and you explain as best you can. Halfway through you ask if it would be better if they took the information direct from your mind. They agree, saying that this would only be done with your permission. They ask for a moment in which they will link themselves together so that all may know and understand. You agree but chuckle silently and wonder if they know what they are letting themselves in for! But it is you who are surprised. The crystals take your deepest most intimate thoughts and mould them into three-dimensional images. Those most deeply hidden erotic desires and dreams of which even you are only dimly conscious are made absolutely clear. You come face to face with your own libido in no uncertain manner.

Your dream of perfect physical love manifests and your whole body reacts to this. You lose all thought of being linked with the crystals, even of being observed, you know only that for you the most erotic and deeply felt act of love is being experienced here and now. As the emotions rise, however, one small area of your mind surfaces and in one illuminating flash of understanding you realize the awesome oneness of the universe, that everything that ever was or has been or will be was there at the beginning, that indeed all life forms are 'starborn'.

As your mind and body move towards a shattering sexual climax you open your whole self not only to the world of crystals but to all life. The response of life is fed back to you through the medium of the crystals, You feel as if your body has shattered into thousands, millions of pieces and each one is a separate being. For one moment in time *you are the universe* at the moment of its creation. You are a part of everything and everything is a part of you, you are totality. Then there is nothing and you drift and dream endlessly through aeons of time until you see in the distance a beautiful green star. It comes nearer and nearer until you can see that it is a doorway made of emerald crystal, with a sapphire eye at its centre. The eye opens and looks at you, the door swings open and you pass through into your own world.

# Ritual 9

# THE CALLING OF A SOUL AND THE HOUSE OF THE GODDESS

## The Programme

The sphere of Binah crowns the Black Pillar of the Tree of Life and is the beginning of form. It has, like all the spheres, many other names: Marah the Great Sea, the Starry Void, the Great Mother, the Bitter Sea, Ama and Aima... All are symbolic of our oceanic cradle, the warm seas of Earth that gave us birth. Binah is irrevocably linked with birth and the beginning of life, but it is also, linked as it is with the planet of Saturn, the giver of death.

All form begins here – not only physical form but its creative and abstract counterparts. Binah is often referred to as the Fount of Faith, for it is from this point on the Tree that all religions, faiths and beliefs emerge. The experience of Binah is said to be that of sorrow, but in giving birth, a woman, providing she is of the maternal type, can also experience great joy and fulfilment.

Most children are born to a welcome, many are not. Some stay only a short while and depart again for the unknown to await another time and place, others do not even draw a breath. Truly Binah holds both joy and sorrow, life and death. Not all who go into the bond of marriage or love partnership desire children – some simply prefer to have each other and the children of the mind. For them the creative urge may lie in the direction of the arts, a chosen and demanding profession, or along whatever life path they have chosen, but for many the blessing of children born from their love and physical union adds perfection and crowns their marriage.

Comparatively few people follow the teachings of the ancient mysteries when compared with the many who do not. Of those, even fewer are privy to the withdrawn teachings concerning love, marriage, physical union and the ritual conception of a child. To go beyond even that and to invoke a special soul to indwell the body ritually prepared for it is to attempt one of the highest and

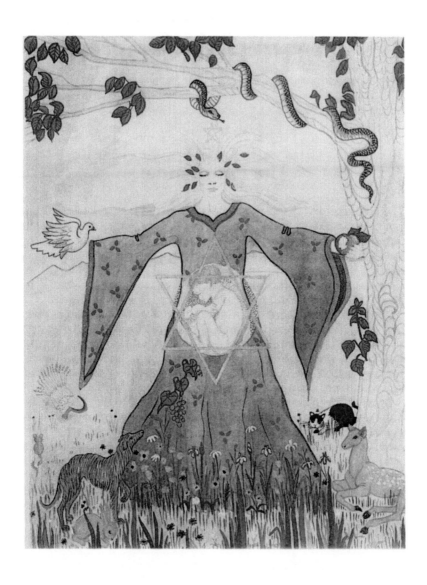

*Figure 20:* The Mother Goddess *(Wolfe van Brussel)*

most heart-rendingly beautiful of all rituals. The keynote of Da'ath, you will remember, was the knowledge of one's divinity. In the Old Testament the knowledge of the Tree of Life was the knowledge of the creative power. To conceive a child is to accept responsibility for another life, a life that may be important to the world in the future, or maybe a life that will one day set off a chain of circumstances that will change history. Or it may simply be a life that will offer love and the promise of your family's immortality through its bloodline. Whichever way you look at it, creating another human being and giving it life is to realize the truth of the Keynote of Da'ath. At this moment initiates working with intent become fully aware of their own divinity. But it is not something to be taken lightly, ever. Binah is also the point of the element of water as Da'ath was the point of the element of highest earth, and from conception the embryo goes through the entire cycle of evolution from life as an aquatic animal to an air breather.

Among the many Goddesses concerned with marriage and childbirth is the Greek Hera, called Juno in the Roman tradition. Strange that she should have been given this area to rule over when her own marriage to Zeus or Jupiter was stormy to say the least. She was not the most motherly of Goddesses and took an instant dislike to her first child, Hephasteus, flinging him from the top of Olympus and injuring the child so badly that he limped forever after. It took many long years before they were reconciled and then only because her son cut her loose after Zeus in a fit of temper chained her across the heavens.

Tuaret, the hippopotamus-headed Goddess of childbirth in the Egyptian tradition was more lovable, and small wooden effigies of her were often found in the tombs of children. In the British Museum there is one sad little 'hippo' toy that has a hinged lower jaw moved by a piece of twisted string, a poignant relic of a much loved child, perhaps carved by the father and laid inside the small sarcophagus to lessen the fear of the long journey towards birth in the new land. The Seven Hathors attended every notable birth and in the case of royal births were said to raise the bed of the queen off the ground so that the new child would be born 'between heaven and earth'. Each Hathor gave the child a gift to mark the occasion of its birth and thus they might well be called the original fairy Godmothers, or the good fairies later to be immortalized in the story of Sleeping Beauty.

Brigid the Celtic fire Goddess was later changed into St Brigit by the early Church Fathers, but tradition says that she was also the Otherworld midwife and was said by some to have presided over the birth of Jesus. The midwife has always been an important part of the magic of childbirth, especially in the Old Tradition. The Hag or Crone was a linking archetype that served at the impregnation

212 THE TREE OF ECSTASY

of the Maiden by the Oak King/Corn King/Horned Lord, according to which particular part of the Craft was followed, and then assisted at the birth of the sun child. Finally, when the sun child became the sacrificed king, it was the Crone who washed his body and laid him out. In this manner birth, life and death have always been part of each other and the three-fold persona of the Great Mother, Binah, Isis, Innana -- call Her by whatever name you will. Even in the Christian religion She has taken up Her old place and is still the Queen of Heaven, Virgin, Mother of the Sun Child, and, at the last, the Stabat Mater, the Mater Dolorosa.

The Mother is perhaps the oldest God form we have. As recounted in the first chapter, even primitive man was awed by the process of birth, and it took a long time before he figured out that it was he who was responsible for the women's fertility. When he did, the Mother was joined by the Horned or Horny/ Erect God. But it was the Mother who was worshipped in the ancient domed temples of the Middle East, made of mud and washed white to reflect the light of both the sun and the moon. Inside on a crudely shaped altar stood the first chalice, the offering of the most precious thing in that desert land, a simple cup of water. The Mother's statues, such as they would have been, were not much advanced from the obese, heavy-breasted, steatopygian figures of the Neanderthal world showing the Fertile Mother, but later would come the slim, chaste, ever virgin Goddesses Diana, Selene, Athena and of course the Undying Isis of a Thousand Names.

To the altars of the Great Mother, and later still to that of the Horned God, came those women who wanted children. In the Delta of the Nile in the small city of Mendes they worshipped a God with a goat's head. In the earliest times the Goat of Mendes was a simple fertility God, the animal's horned head and shaggy nether limbs representing the sexual energy of the most prolific animal the Egyptians knew. Its curving horns emulated the erect male penis and so it became a symbol of the seed-bearer. The God Pan served a similar purpose in ancient Greece. The early Church labelled this simple but incredibly ancient God form 'the Devil', horned and hooved, and consigned it to oblivion except in the remnants of the Old Religion which remembered it only in a debased form. Now it is a symbol so defiled and linked to Satanism that it is impossible to use it even if one wished to do so. Please understand this fully: this particular symbol cannot be used, and those who have the knowledge and the understanding will leave it well alone. I repeat, this symbol cannot be used with safety.

The intention of this ritual is to spiritually prepare both partners, in particular the woman, for conception and for the invoking of the soul that will be housed in the body prepared for it. It is a ritual that not all who use this book will wish to do. If you do not wish to use this ritual, simply leave it out and follow the shorter ritual that follows, the House of the Goddess.

If you intend to work the Calling of a Soul rite, then it is important that you follow the programme exactly if you possibly can. To do this you will have to start some months ahead. Work out the dates when you are mostly likely to conceive, and mark them down. You will also need the help of another woman in the preparation ritual, one who is familiar with the work of the Mysteries and willing to prepare you and your body. Both partners will need to look upon the time of preparation as a build up of pressure on all the levels: on the physical because of the abstinence, on the astral as the partners become aware of the descent of the child's astral body, on the mental as they make contact with the child's psyche and finally on the spiritual as they come into fleeting contact with the Primal Spark and its intermediary, the Individuality, who will 'brief' the new Personality.

Because we have imperfect control over our bodies, it is possible you may not conceive the first time you do the ritual. The particular soul you are invoking may not be ready, your body may not be ready, or the soul may wish to be born into a particular zodiacal energy pattern. Just wait, and when you are ready, do it again. Do not try to force the psyche into a particular gender or type, allow it to manifest as it feels the need. This is an independent *soul* you are inviting, and you have no right to tell it how you want it to manifest, it is a 'come as you are' invitation. The ritual will need an abstinence from sex for one month before it takes place. This will give the womb time to make itself ready and the soul time to make its preparations. It will also allow the man's body to rest and produce a stronger sperm count when the time of conception is right.

The exercises are simple and begin four weeks before the ritual. In addition these weeks should be devoted to cleansing the body from the inside. Cut out all extra rich food, choose fish such as herring and mackerel which are rich in vitamins rather than too much red meat. Eat plenty of fresh vegetables and fruit, and drink at least six pints of water each day, using filtered or bottled water in preference to water from the mains. Cut out all alcohol and if you smoke, this is the time to give it up once and for all – both drinking and smoking can be harmful to the unborn child. Walking and swimming will help to tone the muscles, and take any other form of exercise that you enjoy: golf, tennis, squash, etc. All these things apply to the father as well as the mother, since he provides half the chromosomes. The male half should be as healthy as the female.

A small altar can be set up in the bedroom to the Supernal

Mother and Father and because you are concerned with the first principles of creation it must be very simple. A white cloth, two candles big enough to last for 10 minutes burning morning and evening for the whole four-week period, and a small incense burner will suffice, together with, most importantly, the personal crystals from the last ritual. The candles may be coloured if you wish. That for the Great Mother should be in her colours of black and red, and for the Great Father a pale blue or pale lavender. If required, a small statue of the Great Mother may be used, and the best form to choose would be of Her in Her most primitive shape.

For the first week each evening concentrate on reaching out to the Great Mother for Her help in invoking a soul with whom you already have a strong link. Before sleeping, reach out with the combined strength of your multi-levels to touch, hold and lovingly summon the chosen soul on the highest level. Each morning you will offer a welcome.

As each week passes you will move your powers and your invocations down a level, passing from that of the Primal Spark to the mental where the essence becomes a firm idea, then to the astral where the idea becomes a blueprint, and finally to the physical where conception will take place. This is the inner level pregnancy; that of the physical comes afterwards. Both should be experiences of great worth, beauty and peace.

We start with the first week's exercises. Each evening after bathing, naked, as were our primal parents, sit in meditation before the altar in the candlelight. Synchronize your breathing and relax. Place your hands on the floor in token of the touching of the earth, and in your mind open the chakra just below the feet. Let the earth warmth flow out and start to spin the centre. A thread of light emerges from the middle and moves up to the moon chakra, which opens slowly like a flower. Keep your breathing steady and use it to spin this second centre.

At this point the man holds his moon centre steady but the woman pulls the thread emerging from her centre up to and encircling her sacred chakra so that her womb becomes a still point enclosed within the force of the moon powers. When she feels ready to go on the woman takes the man's hand and they go on, he using the thread from his moon centre and she the thread now coiled around her womb. They let it rise up to the solar chakra and a sudden flare of heat can be felt as the centre begins to spin. In the same way they gradually climb from chakra to chakra until they reach the topmost centre *and emerge beyond their personal Kether*.

Here you pause and find yourselves in the black void that is the womb of the Great Mother. A single star becomes visible and you are drawn towards it until you stand within its brilliance and in the presence of She who holds the keys of life and death. Her voice is all around, wrapping the two of you in silver sounds that become visible to the inner eye as tiny flames and drops of water. A question hangs in the air: 'Why have you come, what do you want of me?'

Now is the time to offer yourselves as a gateway to life. Ask that the chosen soul be one that you have known and loved before so that you may be reunited and continue the journey towards divinity in each other's company. At this point during the first week you may be asked questions, if so *answer with perfect truth*. You may be shown scenes from past lives, if so *watch and wait*. You may be asked to accept a soul who has wronged you and wishes to make amends instead of one you have loved, if so *you must decide*, but not until the last evening's meditation. When the brilliance dims and you find yourselves back in the silent void it is time to retrace your path and close the chakras firmly. Douse the candles and go to bed. On the last evening of this week you will be shown seven spheres, each one shining with a different colour. Allow each one to come close to you and exchange 'emotions', then either choose one soul to come to you or leave the choice to the Great Mother.

In the morning when you wake, lie quietly together and talk over what you saw, felt and heard, then get up, wash, and before eating light the candles and invoke the Great Mother in your own words. Ask for physical plane checks on the information given the night before and for a blessing on your coming ritual. This morning ritual will be the same right through the month.

In the second week follow the same evening meditation path only now when you pass through the personal Kether point you will find yourselves in a world of subtle shifting colours. Wait quietly and there will come to you a sphere of light. If you made your own choice of sphere it will reflect that colour, if you left the choice to a higher authority then simply note the colour for your records. The sphere will come close to you and if you look into it you will see a pattern of shifting energies at its core like minute stars dancing to a complicated rhythm. This is the primal energy pattern of your future child.

On this level (the higher mental) although you may not have noticed it you have the same form, a sphere of light with a dancing energy pattern at its centre. Turn your attention to your partner, observe their pattern and make a note of its movements. Now turn your attention back to the life sphere in front of you, and then turn your sight inwards and observe your own pattern. Because on this highest of mental levels your memory is flawless, you can reproduce an image of those patterns before you. Do it now and look for parts of the pattern that are similar in movement, colour and/or formation. The more similarity you find, the closer the incarnationary or karmic ties there will be between you.

You will also find that you can merge your energy spheres, so try this, the mother first. Slowly and gently, move forward and flow into and around the sphere of your coming child, just as your physical body will enclose its growing form. Proceed slowly and you will find your thought patterns entwining. Old memories may awaken, old ties may be reborn and strengthened. When the contact is strong enough call in the energy sphere of the father so that it envelops mother and child in a protective and loving guardianship. Let the energies and patterns flow in and out of each other, reforging old links and seeding new ones. Do not spend too long together the first time, it can be draining to stay at this level. The father separates first, then the mother. Withdraw slowly and don't be sad, soon you will be together for a another lifetime. Do this exercise each night for the second week and follow the usual morning procedure.

The third week's evening exercise will follow the same path but now to the level of the high astral. Each succeeding week the essence of the child will be drawn lower and lower until during the actual ritual it will be poised above the vortex of creative power set up and maintained by the physical union of the parents. This vortex will be kept open and steady by the repeating of the sexual union morning and evening on three successive days. This will give both sperm and ova the maximum chance of uniting. The Mysteries pertaining to the sacred marriage teach that every part of the human body has a minute portion of consciousness, therefore, say the teachings, when a sacred marriage is performed and its ritually inspired consummation is directed towards the birth of a child, the ova is able to summon to itself the one sperm among millions that is destined to complete the unity.

When your consciousness opens on to the astral level it will feel as if you are swimming in a warm sea. You can see no horizon and so the astral matter surrounds and upholds you in a misty hazy landscape. Shapes and forms, human, animal and abstract, appear and disappear, some lasting a few moments, others longer. Colours shift and grow deeper or lighter, sounds echo back to you from unseen voices. All these are your thoughts continually becoming, changing and evolving. Try to keep your mind fixed on one object and see how long you can keep it in that form. It is surprisingly difficult and will depend on your ability to concentrate – something you learned long ago in your occult training, or should have done!

You can feel your partner near you and suddenly there is another form, unseen but felt and known. Your child has moved a level nearer to the physical plane. The form is that of an adult and is androgynous, for as yet the soul has not decided which sex will offer the better opportunities for the soul to evolve. Take turns in holding your child, assuring the soul of your love and desire for its full manifestation. Now come together, arms entwined. Tell the soul of your hopes for its new life, keep reassuring it of a welcome. It can be a frightening thing to approach a new birth and very few will have this kind of welcome, even those who are wanted. Each partner should give the other some time alone with the child, then they should all come together again just before leaving. At the last speak of the sexual vortex you will soon create to act as a doorway into the physical world. This will help to allay any fears the soul may have. Perhaps you may like to give it a sign to follow, a ring of flowers at the mouth of the vortex, a 'welcome mat' so to speak. Each night you will draw closer to your coming child. It may speak of hopes and fears for the future – try to remember them. It will try to cling to you, but reassure it and gently withdraw until the next night. Follow the usual instructions for the following morning.

Now comes the last week of preparation. Follow the same path but as you pass beyond the last chakra you will come into what can only be described as the Earth of the visionary. You will see your usual surroundings but as they really are in the delicate colours and full grace of their ideal form. Trees, flowers, gardens, rooms and even furniture will glow and the molecular structure that holds them in the Earth level will be seen clearly. When you look at each other you will see yourselves as you truly are, beings destined for Godhood, and also two people drawing closer to a fulfilment of their physical union. The female genital centre is iridescent, like a dragonfly's wing, and just above it the sacred chakra of the womb looks like a pearl with a deep rose-coloured centre. The whole aura of the male is the Yesodic violet, with the genital area slightly lighter in colour. The life-engendering sperm can be clearly seen within the testicles like pin-points of light.

Breathe regularly and deeply and in rhythm with each other. Visualize the journey of the sperm and its joining with the ova in a tiny flash of light. From the established foetus a tiny thread of light emerges and links itself to the sacred centre of its mother. The future mother should envisage her womb as a resting place for the child-to-be. Think of its warmth and safety and the steady growth of the child. The future father should concentrate on his role as guardian of both mother and child and see them together within the protecting ring of his aura. Now change over, with the mother seeing and feeling herself as the female protector of her family, its strength in time of need and trouble. The father should visualize himself as the child's source of food, love and attention. In this way the idea is planted of both parents being protectors and cherishers, sharing their roles instead of each sex sticking to their stereotypes.

Also during the third week there are two minor rituals to be performed, one for the woman and one for the man. Both are performed on consecutive days with the help of the female friend in place of the usual evening exercise. The first one is for the two women. Prepare a small altar with white cloth and scatter it with flower petals. On it place a lighted candle, a small incense burner with incense already burning, some water and salt mixed together, a small bottle of anointing oil and a chalice of wine. The woman comes to the altar clothed only in a white sheet or a white robe. Her friend acts as priestess. The woman kneels before the altar and offers a posy of flowers.

*Priestess:* You come before the altar of the Great Mother to ask for the blessing of a child and to be cleansed in the ancient manner to prepare yourself to house a new soul. Speak now and ask what you desire of She who is the mother of all that has lived and that will live in the future.

*Woman:* I ask that I and the man of my heart and my choice may be blessed in our lives by the presence of a soul known and loved in the past that we may again live and grow together. Therefore I offer my body to the will of the Great Mother and ask Her for this gift of new life. I come willingly to be cleansed and made ready. Let the appointed soul know that it will be welcomed and loved.

*She stands and takes off the robe to stand naked before the altar. The priestess takes the salt and water and sprinkles it on the woman's head, hands and feet, then marks the womb with the pentacle symbol.*

*Priestess:* Woman, I make thee clean and sweet before the Goddess with salt and water to clear away all that has no place in thee.

*She takes up the censer and censes her.*

With the smoke of incense I make thee sacred and a fitting chalice for life.

*She marks her with oil on the head, hands, feet and womb, using the crescent symbol.*

With oil I hallow thee and the womb within thy body. Let it be filled with life from the seed of the man of thy choice, if that shall be the will of the Mother.

*She gives her wine from the chalice then marks her womb with a pentacle in wine, and also her hands and feet.*

The chalice is the Mother, in the wine is the seed of the Horned One, together they shall prepare thee for the holding of life.

*She gives her the candle to hold.*

With light in thy hand, in thy mind, in thy heart and in thy womb, do you offer yourself as a chalice for a new life?

*Woman:* I do offer myself as a chalice. In token of this I offer one drop of my blood to the chalice.

*She offers her hand to the priestess who pricks it with a new needle and allows one drop to enter the wine-filled cup.*

*Priestess:* Then so shall it be. The Goddess accepts your offer and grants your request.

*She offer the chalice to the woman who upends the candle and douses it in the wine. She must then drink the wine to the dregs.*

*Priestess:* It is done. The womb is prepared, the soul has been summoned.

On the following evening it will be the turn of the male partner. It is essential that the woman acting as priestess be known and trusted by him and that he feels comfortable being naked in her presence. The altar is prepared as before and the man comes to it clothed only in a robe and barefoot. He kneels to offer a small amount of (pure) honey to the altar.

*Priestess:* You are before the altar of the Great Mother. What do you want of her?

*Man:* I would ask that She who holds the gift of life and death fills my seed with the fire of life that I may fill the womb chalice of the woman who holds my heart. With her I wish to create a physical body to house a soul drawn to us by love.

*Priestess:* Will you serve the Goddess in the body of the human woman? For such a mating as this was in ancient times called the Rite of Nuit. The Goddess Herself, invoked by the power of love, will descend into the chosen woman and you will mate with both the woman you love and the Great Mother Herself, as did Osiris when the young jackal was conceived to become the guide and teacher of mankind. Will you give your seed to the Goddess in the woman, so that the woman in the Goddess may bring forth?

*Man:* I will give my seed to the Goddess.

*He takes off his robe to stand naked before the altar. The priestess takes the salt and water and sprinkles it over his head, hands, penis and feet.*

*Priestess:* I shall make thee clean and sweet before the Goddess and wash away all that has no place in thee.

*She takes the censer and censes him.*

With the smoke of incense I shall make thee sacred and fit to mate with the Goddess.

*She anoints him with honey on his mouth, hands and penis.*

With honey I make thee sweet and the force within thee strong.

*She gives him one sip from the chalice and traces a pentacle on his belly with wine.*

Wine is the blood of the Gods. May the ancient one, he of the horn, fill you with his power.

*Man:* I pray that this shall be so.

*He steps forward, takes the candle and the chalice, bows to the priestess, douses the candle in the wine and drinks it down.*

*Priestess:* As the candle and the flame is to the God, so the chalice and the wine is to the Goddess. Together they shall create new life.

*Both:* So shall it be. The soul will be summoned.

For the rest of the week the evening exercise will consist of a repeat of an earlier exercise where the woman sits on a chair covered with a blue or green cloth, naked and crowned with flowers. The man sits at her feet and concentrates on seeing her as the Garment of the Goddess. He should look at her face and body, hair and skin, her eyes and expression, see the Great Mother mirrored there and praise Her as the giver of both life and death. The following evening the roles should be reversed. Do this to the end of the week and the night of the full ritual.

# The Calling of a Soul

## Sphere = Binah. Keynote = The Power of Two to Become Three.

*To prepare your place of worship first clean the room thoroughly and take out anything that is not needed as far as is possible. Cover the bed with a new sheet, and then cover the sheet with flowers and sweet herbs of every kind. Place a chalice of wine and a small plate of biscuits near the bed. Light the room with candles only and cense it with incense before using it, in addition to the ritual preparation you will find in Chapter 6 for the preparation of a sacred place. Fill the room with flowers, for you are preparing to welcome a guest.*

*The robe for the woman should be a deep blue and should open down the front completely. That of the man should be light blue and fold over, tied with a cord. Both should be barefoot. Eat sparingly before the rite, bathe carefully, paying attention to hair, nails, feet and especially to the sexual parts – they must be scrupulously clean. No perfumes should be used on the body at all. The incense should be light and unobtrusive. If music is used it must not be strident and it must be kept low. The Mother's altar should have a small light on it and nothing else.*

*Hand in hand the two come before the altar. They offer a prayer to the Great Mother.*

*Both:* Thou who art the giver of life and death be with us this night, be our canopy of stars, our moon, and our guide. Breathe into us thy divine breath and fill us with light. If it be thy will may the rite be fruitful and the fruit itself perfect in form and mind. So mote it be.

*The man turns and calls the Goddess into the woman. He places his hand upon her head.*

Man: Thee I invoke, lady of love and beauty. Enter into this physical garment prepared for thee.

*He opens her robe and kisses her breast.*

Enter into the heart that adores thee in thy majesty.

*He opens her robe further and kisses her womb.*

Enter into the sacred centre, cleansed and made holy to receive both the physical body and the immortal soul, if it be thy will.

*He opens her robe fully and kisses her pudenda.*

Enter into the cave of stars that I may be surrounded by thy divine presence on entering the sacred chamber of life.

*He rises.*

*The woman discards her robes completely then invokes the Horned God upon the man. (If you are diffident about using a Horned God image then replace the horns in your visualization with curving rays of light such as were seen upon the head of Moses when he came down from the Mount.) She places her hand upon his head.*

Woman: Thee I invoke, the fiery power of the life force, the great giver of the seed of stars.

*She opens his robe and kisses his breast.*

Enter into the heart that yearns to receive thee in thy full strength.

*She opens his robe further and kisses his navel.*

Enter into the belly of thy priest and fill him with thy divine vigour.

*She opens his robe fully and kisses his penis.*

Enter into the rod of life, take thy priest unto thyself and in joining with me, join with the Great Goddess, Mother of all that breathes and lives.

*Wait for the divine forces to enter. Help them by building up the forms within the heart centre and allowing them to grow until they almost fill the physical body. At this point in the ritual the man and the woman become actual vehicles for the Goddess and the God. The God leads his Goddess to the prepared bed and lays her down. Taking some oil in his hands he begins to massage and caress her body, deliberately arousing her sexually as he does so. After a little while the Goddess does the same for him. The more sensuous the touch, the greater the preparation of the bodies to give and to receive the life force. Do not neglect words, for the voice and the language of love can be powerful aphrodisiacs. Praise your partner's body, and his/her response to touch and stimulation. Speak of the child whose body you are planning to create and the soul you hope will enter it. Speak of the pleasure and happiness you will experience in the carrying of this precious child, a symbol of your love, or of seeing the woman growing round and full like the moon and knowing it is your child she carries. This time is special and should not be rushed. Allow the sexual tide to rise as slowly as you can: the slower it rises, the greater will be the power of the vortex you will create between you.*

*Call the child by name if you have chosen one, or by a 'baby' name. Ask the soul to be ready to enter the vortex. Whatever sexual position you favour best should be used and when the power is so great that it cannot be held back the joining begins. As the phallus enters the vagina the Calling of the Soul begins. In the silence of the heart let the man and the woman, the God and the Goddess, begin to open the vortex.*

*The woman's invocation:*

To the will of the Great Goddess I open my heart and my sacred centre. I call to my child beyond the vortex of the life power, I summon the soul of my future child and bid it enter that vortex unafraid and in the knowledge of love and welcome. With gentleness I will receive thee and with strength I will surround thee. My blood shall nourish thee and my flesh shall provide for thee. In the soft darkness of my womb I will hold thee safe and bring thee to the light. I am the gateway to the world, enter and rest. Blessed be the man who entrusts his seed to me and blessed be the child whose body springs from the Rite of Nuit.

*The man's invocation:*

To the ancient God of the Horn I open my heart that the power of life shall be with me. Let the seed that springs from me be pure and unblemished, that the coming soul may have a perfect vehicle in which to dwell. I call my child from beyond the void, I summon the soul with love and with joy. With my strength I shall guard and cherish thee. My flesh and my blood I share with thee. Blessed be this woman who is the chalice to my seed, and blessed be the child that comes from the chalice.

*Try to remain fully conscious of the culmination of the rite and at that moment visualize the great vortex above you and the descent of the soul into the womb. Try to see with the eyes of the spirit the downpouring of grace and light that comes with a soul that is ritually invoked. This is a mating that occurs on four levels: the physical, the astral, the mental and the spiritual. At the moment of sexual climax the way is open from the highest level to the lowest and the descent is made.*

*Rest now, and sleep. It may be that the power of the vortex will draw you into its centre again before morning, if so, follow its pull and fill the chalice again. During your sleep the charged essences of the Goddess and the God will leave you and all will be accomplished.*

# The House of The Goddess

This is an alternative ritual for those that do not wish to invoke for a child. However the foregoing ritual can also be used to invoke for a 'child of the mind', i.e. a development that might truly be called a 'brain-child'.

The 'House' referred to in this ritual is the priestess, for in ancient times a woman who dedicated herself to one aspect of the Goddess for life was seen as a dwelling-place for the Goddess. Hence the term 'the Garment of Isis' given to certain priestesses of that aspect of the Great Mother. To refer to them as temple prostitutes is quite wrong and shows a total misconception of their function. They were trained to move their conscious selves to one side and to allow the Goddess to indwell for a space of time. This is what modern occultists would term 'mediation' as opposed to mediumship, and it enables the seer to maintain consciousness on two and even three levels at the same time.

At certain times of the year a chosen priest would become the consort of Isis through the mediatorship of her priestess. The *hieros gamos* or sacred marriage was to them a very real and deeply religious undertaking, and this ritual should be seen in the same light, for it is based on a similar theme.

*The altar is dressed in black and silver with three white or silver candles, a censer with burning incense, a small amount of pure honey, anointing oil and three red roses. The priestess is dressed in black or white and her robe should open down the front. The priest is in white or grey/blue, and his robe should also open fully. The bed is prepared as for the Calling of a Soul.*

*The priestess takes her place behind the altar, the priest before it. He lights the incense and then the first candle.*

*Priest:* Hail to thee, Isis, Queen of Heaven and Earth, the temple awaits thy footstep.

*He lights the second candle.*

Hail to thee who is beauty incarnate, Daughter of Nuit, hail.

*He lights the third candle.*

Hail Sothis, star of Egypt, giver of life and death, mother of Horus the Avenger. Lady of magic, hail.

*The priestess should visualize the descent of Isis upon her, covering her like a silver veil.*[1]

*When aware of the presence of the Goddess, she speaks:*

*Priestess:* The call is answered and the Goddess comes. She has

---

[1] The actual assumption of a God form I have dealt with in *The Ritual Magic Workbook* (The Aquarian Press, 1986).

taken on her garment and sets foot upon the earth. He who would claim that garment must prove himself worthy to wear it.

*The priest comes round the altar, takes the priestess/Isis by the hand and leads her round to the front of the altar. He takes the incense and censes her three times to each side and three times from head to foot.*

*Priest:* I offer incense to thy right side and bid thee welcome. I offer incense to thy left side and bid thee welcome. I offer incense to thy head and adore thy wisdom, to thy body and adore thy beauty, to thy feet and beg thee to stay that I may honour thee.

*He takes the honey and places a little on her tongue.*

With honey I make my name sweet upon thy lips, and like the honey bee I take it from thee.

*He kisses her. Then he takes the oil, rubs it between her breasts, and kisses them.*

Let me adorn the beauty of thy breasts with perfume and rest between them.

*He rubs oil into the palms of her hands and kisses them.*

I shall perfume your hands that they may caress me and fill me with their scented gentleness.

*He rubs oil into her pudenda and kisses it.*

I will honour the cave of stars with perfume and let its fragrance go before me that I may enter like unto a king in majesty. Enroyal me, Great Isis, empower me and call me Pharaoh of the Two Lands. Place me in thy lap, feed me from thy breast and make me immortal in thy sight.

*Priestess/Isis:* You shall be my lord and love, King of the Two Lands for the time of our coming together, for in me Egypt is present here. You shall lie upon the breast of Isis and breathe her breath. Between her breasts you will become the Pharaoh, mighty in power, yet before her power weak like a child. The sceptre of earthly power sinks down before Isis.

*He takes the roses from the altar and 'Isis' leads him to the 'royal couch' and opens his robe.*

*Priestess/Isis:* On thy right breast I kiss thee, on thy left breast I kiss thee and now rises your kingly strength. On thy belly I kiss thee and the heat of the sun rises in thee. On thy phallus I kiss thee and claim thee as my Osiris.

*The priest lays his Isis down and places the head of the first rose between her breasts and the second over the sacred centre before scattering the petals of the last rose over the triangle of her womanhood.*

*Priest:* Queen, Goddess and love, I salute thee. Open the gate of kingship to me that I may enter and with thy power of enroyalment claim my kingdom. Without thee I am but a man. In thee is the sceptre raised and the Nile shall flood, bringing joy to the land.

*'Isis' calls her priest to her in the ancient way and the sexual power*

*generated between them causes the astral Nile to rise and flood the land of Egypt, represented by Isis herself. The river has always flooded the fields as the star of the Goddess rises, and for centuries has kept the land fertile and fed the people. This ritual symbolizes the flooding and would have been enacted by the Pharaoh and the high priestess each year.*

*When the sexual climax has been reached and both have recovered they must return to the altar to give thanks.*

*Priest:* The land has been saved and the power of Isis has been shown to the people. I have become Osiris and I shall rise again and bless my people with corn. Hail to thee, Isis, Queen of Heaven, Star of the South. Blessed be thy name eternally.

*Priestess/Isis:* I am Egypt, I am woman and Goddess, I am Isis, I am all things to all men. I shall endure to the end of time and beyond. A blessing shall rest upon she who is my garment, and upon this house wherein the ancient rite has been recalled.

*The woman now releases the Isis power and the lights are put out. It is important that both sleep as soon as possible to restore the energy that this ritual can require of the mind and body.*

# The Pathworking

You are walking on the shore of a warm sea, your bare feet lapped by little waves that kiss and run. It is night and the sky is lit with millions of bright stars like fireflies pinned to a black curtain. You pause and stand looking out at the restless sea. You too are restless, waiting for something, but you do not know what you are waiting for except that the very thought of it makes your breath halt in your throat and your limbs tremble. Everything around is hushed and poised on the edge of an experience, the night birds have fallen silent, the wind has dropped, even the sea seems to have become motionless. This is the time of the uttermost ebb when the sea pauses before turning her tides.

Your eyes are drawn to the horizon, the very edge where sea and sky merge into one indeterminate existence. You see a flash of light there, and again. A third time it flashes and then becomes steady: it is the moon. Slowly and majestically she rises in her fullness from the ocean, lingering for a second as her rim leaves the sea for the sky, then she is climbing higher and higher.

Far out to sea a bright light moves on the water. It comes nearer and nearer, and gradually becomes a shape, a woman, tall and straight as a tree. She walks just below the surface of the sea and it foams around her like a lace edging to her gown of silver grey and white. Her hair streams out behind her like a cloud of black silk, here and there a star gleams through its raven lustre echoing the star that shines on her high clear forehead. Her form is lissom and has the ripeness of youth. Through the thin silk of her robe her nipples appear like delicate pink flowers. A girdle of pearl and amber clasps a waist as supple as a willow and her breath perfumes the air about you.

Slowly you look up into her face and meet the lustrous eyes. She is radiant like the moon itself. Her skin gleams with the lustre of pearl and her dark eyes settle gently upon you, seeming to question why you are here. The pressure of the Goddess' presence is too much and you sink to your knees, knowing only that you must adore and worship this being with everything that is in you This is the maiden aspect of the Goddess, Her virgin girdle as yet unloosed, emerging from the sea of Her birth. She passes by, Her footprints too light to be seen on the sand. For a moment She pauses and the gentle touch of Her hand is felt upon your head, and the murmured blessing flows over your soul like balm easing the hurts of life away and leaving only joy. Then She passes on her way.

The scene changes and you are walking in a ripe cornfield. It is noon and the sun shines down with just the hint of a breeze to cool its fire. In the heat the birdsong is slow and lazy and even the small river edging the field with blue and silver seems to flow more slowly. The corn is wounded here and there with the blood-red colour of poppies and all is silent in the heat of the day. A tree stands in the centre of the field and offers welcome shade and fruit to ease your thirst. You climb up into the branches to pluck the best and settle down to rest cradled by the intersecting boughs that bear you up as easily as a child. Half-asleep, you drowse and drift.

Her laughter brings you awake, you turn in your leafy bed and look down. Coming through the corn is a woman, it is She, the Lady of the Sea, only now Her hair is golden and Her eyes bluer than the cornflowers – but you would know Her anywhere. Her robe is golden brown, the colour of sun-baked earth and held on Her shoulder with a pin of amber and gold. Her laughter echoes in the stillness of the sun-drenched field as She runs from the tall figure that follows Her.

A match for Her in beauty of face and form, the corn king pursues Her and runs Her to ground under the tree. Laughing, She sinks to the ground and allows him his fill of kisses. Suddenly the birdsong seems more intense, the heat more sultry and from the wood on a nearby hill there comes the sound of pipes. Pan is here.

Below you the oldest of all stories is being acted out, the amber pin is removed and the earth-gold robe falls away. The Goddess form beneath is full and tempting, her breasts rounded and demanding the homage of her consort's lips. The dappled awning offered by the tree drapes her in a robe of light and shade, entrancing and provocative. The curve of belly and thigh is the dream of a sculptor and his despair at ever copying its perfection. The darker gold that hides and yet proclaims Her womanhood has been covered with scarlet petals, poppies that gladly give their colour for Her adornment.

The corn king's time is now, for the Earth Goddess is his to claim, and claim Her he does in all his strength and power. The scarlet of poppy is joined by the scarlet of a new found pain and joy and above and around it all is the high sweet piping urging them on.

You feel no shame in watching the mating of the Goddess and her king, for it is for you and all humanity that this is done to feed the land and its growth. To mate is natural, beautiful and ordained by The One as an eternal gift for God and human alike. Your eyes are heavy and the two figures below you are silent now. Slowly your eyes close and you dream, dream of a king laughing even as the flash of silver gleams above him.

The sun passes on towards its setting and you open your eyes. Below you lies the corn king smiling in his deepest sleep. A scarlet drift of poppies covers him and in his heart is the amber pin. The seed-filled Goddess has gone and will bear the corn king renewed in the fullness of time, for this is Her mother aspect.

All changes again and you are lying on a grassy hill. Above the night sky is filled with stars. In the branches of a tall tree a new moon hangs, caught like a white bird in flight. The sounds of the night are all about you and as you look up the stars seem to gather and form a face. It is the face of a woman, the Goddess, lovely but older, sad yet smiling. Her hair flows like silver across the night sky, Her eyes hold all the wisdom of the Earth and stars and beyond. She is time and change, youth and age, cruel and loving. She is maiden and mother and wise woman, she is the Goddess, Binah the Bitter Sea, Aphrodite and Demeter, Persephone and Hecate. She is all things and never-ending. But you must wake.

# Ritual 10

# THE ADORATION OF THE PILLAR

## The Programme

As the cup, the cauldron, the circle and the *vesica pisces* have always been seen as symbols for the female womb and vulva, so the wand, the rod, the tree and the pillar have symbolized the male penis in the state of erection. As the last ritual was centred in and around the mothering aspect of the woman, so this ritual will be for the fathering aspect of the man. World mythology abounds in legends of the male Gods descending to mate with the daughters of men. Indeed it can be found in the Bible set out in plain words: '. . . and the Sons of God looked upon the daughters of men and saw that they were fair, and took to wife such as they chose' (Genesis 6:2).

The exploits of Zeus and his many amours with human women are a well-known part of classical Greek mythology, and he was by no means the only one: Apollo, Ares, Hermes, Poseidon and Hades all fathered children on human mothers. Since there is always a basic kernel of truth in every myth we must assume there was an original purpose in these God/human sexual relationships. There is of course the old stand-by explanation that the Gods were stranded extraterrestrials who tried to blend into the human race by passing on their bloodline to children fathered on native stock. Or such myths could simply be a way of expunging from the racial subconscious the memory of the 'Mother' taking the strongest and most successful hunter to her bed to bear children from his superior genetic stock. Or it might be a garbled folk-memory of an unknown but more advanced tribe overrunning and conquering a native people – the most efficient way of establishing one's claim is to breed into the conquered race and at the same time deny the native males access to their own women.

The hard, rending and penetrating shape of the phallus became a symbol of the fighting male, the warrior and conqueror. H.Cutner, in his book *A Short History of Sex Worship*, states:

The word phallus may have taken its origin from a Semitic word palash or palas, meaning to break through, or press into . . . in the Sanscrit it is phal, phalla, or phul . . . and has the meaning of a fully ripe fruit ready to eject the seed it contains.

As time went on and the worship of the male God(s) fully superseded that of the female Goddess, the setting up of stone pillars for the purpose of worship increased throughout the Mediterranean cultures. Some of these bore the sculpted head and shoulders of a God, either Pan or Priapus, and were called Herms. They were often set up by the roads along which pilgrims travelled to and from the temples. This scandalized the early Christians who saw the Herms as obscene, but in its origin the worship of sex was pure in its intention, practised by those who saw nothing in its rites but praise to that which kept the earth filled with life.

The single standing stone so often found throughout Europe is a phallic symbol par excellence and very often if the area around it is investigated it will be found that around the stone there appears to be a vortex of force. When these two symbols are translated we have the feminine vortex with its spinning power penetrated by the rigid masculine power, both being pinned as it were to the earth and thereby bringing it new life.

The following ritual has as its intention the adoration of the fire of life as symbolized by the sacred pillar, the lingam, the phallus. By concentrating the attention and intention upon the male symbol it calls on the life force ever present in the universe and forces it to descend into the organ prepared for it. It acts in a similar way to the last ritual where a soul was contacted and a physical vessel prepared for its descent via the vortex of force set by the sexual act. Therefore this ritual may well cause a marked increase in the male's sexual interest in the week prior to the ritual and in actual sexual activity during the week following the ritual.

During the ritual the male plays a somewhat passive role at first and only manifests the 'fire' of the pillar of life towards the end. The female's role is that of the Goddess Ma'at who, so legend states, was manifest before the Gods themselves and even before creation. This ritual can be worked either indoors or outside. If the latter then I suggest it be on a warm summer's evening when twilight is falling.

The God form used for the male partner is one of the earliest in Egyptian legend: Atum-Ra. He is sometimes depicted as being lion-headed. It is said of him that he created the world and then brought the first Gods into being by masturbating into his clenched fist.

He was the lord of both order and chaos and superimposed one upon the other to bring the world into being, then used his own

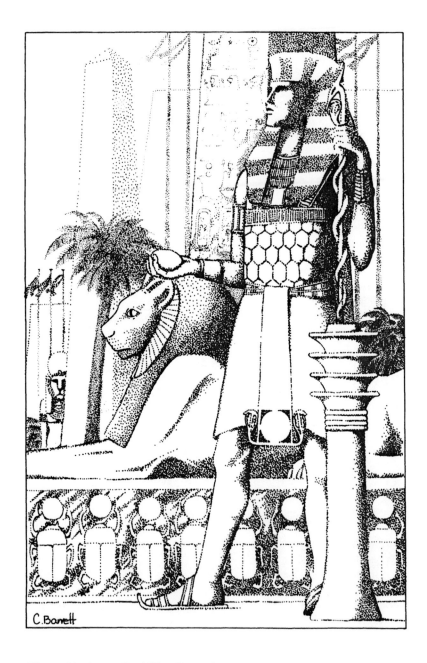

*Figure 21:* **Atum-Ra** *(Clive Barrett)*

seed to give life to Tefnut and Shu, the first male and female Gods. The Egyptians had quite a few ithyphallic Gods, among them Min the God of fertility, Ptah the God of life, and Khnum the potter God who created physical bodies on his potter's wheel.

The symbols best used for meditation are the stone phallus or any phallic shape. (A stone or wooden phallus was sometimes used in certain cultures to break through the virginity of a bride before she went to her marriage bed. This was done because it was believed that the blood shed on the breaking of the hymen could cause sterility and impotence in the bridegroom. Sometimes a slave was used as a substitute for the husband. This practice is still in existence in a few places.) Other symbols for use would be a simple stone pillar, a tau cross or a pine cone atop a rod – this latter is the basis of the Bacchic sceptre called a thyrsus.

As you will already have made a lingam/yoni altar-piece for the third ritual you will already have something on which to meditate and use for the altar afterwards.

The morning exercise for the male partner is as follows. On waking stretch the body gently and slowly until the muscles are flexible. You will need a bath towel or folded blanket laid out on the floor. If the room is warm enough then take off any night-clothes you may be wearing. Lie down on your back and take up a star position with your arms and legs stretched out. Open the head chakra, visualizing it as a sphere of golden light enclosing the top half of the head. Stabilize the sphere and then push out of its right side a beam of golden light going down towards your hand on that side. Build up a smaller sphere of light enclosing the hand. Now push out another beam of light going towards the right foot and make another sphere, then cross over to the left foot and so on. Continue in this way until you have formed a pentagon of light all around yourself. Build up the power at each contact point and send up a beam of light from each one, bending them to meet and form another sphere placed just above the sexual centre (see Fig 22). Use this sphere to draw down power from your Higher Self and use that power to energize the centre. By using this ring of auric power to encircle the body and call down your own higher spiritual power you create a self-perpetuating flow of power that will vitalize any centre towards which it is directed.

The female partner can use the same exercise, concentrating the power on the triangle formed by her hands and genitals. To close down, simply dismiss the central sphere, allow the beams from the contact points to retract, and then wind up the power in the reverse direction, starting from the left side of the head and moving round. Allow 15 to 20 minutes minimum for this exercise.

For the evening exercise, sit in contemplation of the lingam

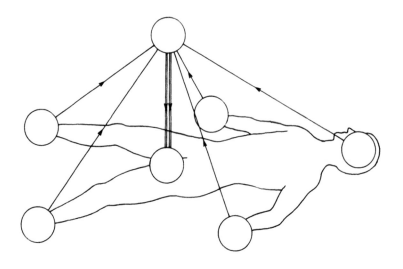

*Figure 22:* Drawing down power from the Higher Self

symbol with a burning candle before, behind and at each side of
you so that you are surrounded by light. This applies to both
partners. For the ritual itself you will need to prepare the bed as
before, if you are working indoors. If you are outside then a
sleeping bag or thick blanket will do. You will also need a throne
for the 'Atum'. If indoors this can be a chair covered with a sheet
and decorated with flowers and perhaps a piece of deep blue cloth
thrown across the back. If out of doors then a rock or fallen tree
can suffice if treated in the same way. The Atum wears a simple
Egyptian headdress (see Fig 23), but is otherwise nude. If you
have the skill to make replicas of the crook and flail symbols they
would be very appropriate. Ma'at can wear the robe used for Isis
in the Resurrection of Osiris.

   On either side of the throne place bowls of fruit, flowers and/or
plants – anything that can symbolize life in all its many forms. A
small table will serve as an altar to one side. It should carry
incense, an Ankh, a chalice with pure spring water, and a small
piece of bread, homemade of coarse flour if possible, with a small
bowl of honey. There must also be a piece of silk – real silk – about
the size of a small towel or scarf, and a jar of oil, with lastly a pot
half filled with sweet earth, some extra earth ready, and some
seeds or bulbs for planting.

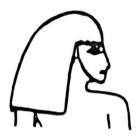

*Figure 23:* An Egyptian headdress

Some music is appropriate during this ritual and I would suggest a tape of unaccompanied harp music, or, if it is possible, some tapes of music for Egyptian ritual – they should be available from a good occult supply shop. Failing this, try some of Bob Stewart's exquisite psaltery music.

If working indoors, draw the curtains and prepare enough candles around the room to give a comfortable light, but at the beginning light just one in the far corner of the room.

# The Adoration of the Pillar

## Sphere = Chocmah. Keynote = The Masculine Engendering Power.

*As soon as it gets dark the rite may begin. The Atum enters and takes his place on the throne. He meditates on the Manifestation of Life for some time. Ma'at enters and takes her place on a cushion by the altar. The music begins, but very softly. Atum speaks:*

*Atum:* I behold the manifestation of earth and heaven out of chaos. Night and day have I, Atum, Lord of Creation, wrought out of the darkness of the unmade. Now I will rest. *(Pauses, as if in thought.)* Yet it is not in my nature to rest and there is within my heart an emptiness, for there is no other with whom I can share my existence. I call to the Gods who exist beyond such as I, and ask for deliverance from my loneliness.

*Ma'at:* I hear a voice in the darkness, a voice of despair. It calls upon those Gods beyond the Gods who have outlived time itself. Such a one am I, Ma'at, Goddess of Truth and of Absolute Justice.

*She lights one candle in the far corner.*

THE TREE OF ECSTASY

Behold, Lord of Creation, I give you hope. Ask of me three questions and I will answer truthfully.

*Atum:* Goddess of the Far Beyond, I ask this question: how can I end my solitary vigil over that which I have created?

*Ma'at:* By creating others like yourself, and by giving them that greatest of all powers, the ability to love and give birth to others of their kind. That is my answer to your first question.

*She lights another candle.*

*Atum:* Tell me how I may create others of my own kind, for that is a mystery hidden from me.

*Ma'at:* The pillar of life and the secret it holds lies between the thighs of Atum Ra, creator of the world. With this and with the womb of a woman you can create others like yourself. That is my answer to your second question.

*She lights another candle.*

*Atum:* In all creation there is no woman with whom I can create life. How can I find such a one?

*Ma'at:* Atum, you hold her within you: she is your inner and higher self, your divine mate sleeping in your heart. She needs only to be awakened. Put your right hand into your left side and you will touch the womb of your higher self. Bring it forth into the light and guard it gently in your hand. Fill it with fire from the pillar between your thighs and the woman will come forth from you to live with you and bring the fire to life. She will never leave you but will stay to guide the Gods and humanity to the Gods beyond time. This is my answer to your third question.

*She lights all the candles.*

*Atum:* I have heard thy wisdom and I shall awaken my higher self.

*He puts down his crook and flail, places his right hand on his left side and withdraws it as a clenched fist which he now places over his heart.*

Behold, Goddess of Truth, it is done. How it flutters in my hand, like a small bird caught in a net. Fear not, I shall hold thee gently and fill thee with the fire of my love. Together we shall bring the Gods to birth and you shall sit beside me and give me your counsel in all things.

*Ma'at:* Thy woman self stirs and wakens. Her power grows and calls to thee. Hers shall be the first form to issue from her own womb and her name shall be called Tefnut. With thee she shall create her brother Shu. From these three shall all others come forth. I shall prepare thee.[1]

*She brings incense and censes Atum.*

*Ma'at:* With perfumed incense I prepare thee.

---

[1] I am aware that Tefnut was the daughter only of Atum, and have used my prerogative of poetic licence to make her sister, wife, and daughter in this ritual.

*She returns the incense, brings the Ankh and holds it to the nose of Atum.*

With the scent of life I fill thy nostrils, O Atum.

*She returns the Ankh, brings the water and sprinkles it over Atum's head and penis.*

With pure water I wash thee.

*She returns the water, brings the bread and honey and places a piece on his tongue.*

With honey I sweeten thy mouth and feed thy inner self.

*She returns the bread and takes up the silk which she brings to Atum and places on his lap beneath the phallus. Then she kneels before him and taking up the oil pours just a little into her hands. She takes the phallus of Atum between her palms. Atum must remain with his clenched fist over his heart, silent and without moving until Ma'at directs him to move.*

Ma'at: The pillar of Atum shall rise and be filled with the fire of life. I shall call forth from him that which shall be his guide and counsel and live in his heart forever.

*She gently caresses and encourages the penis to a full erection, then salutes it with her lips.*

May the pillar of life live forever. May the fire within never die. May Atum, Lord of Life, find peace on the breast of Tefnut the firstborn.

*She takes the silk and wraps it around the erect penis, then, taking Atum's hand from his breast, clasps it around the silk, with her hand over his.*

Let the fire leap from the pillar. Let the womb of thy hand be filled. Atum, bring life into the world that has been created.

*Together the two Gods bring the fire and the seed from Atum. He must strive to keep everything but the intention of the ritual from his mind, for it must be offered to the power of creation. When it has been accomplished Atum takes up his crook and flail again. Ma'at takes the semen-filled scarf, places it in the prepared earth and covers it with more earth, then sprinkles it with the seeds. Alternatively if you have a garden it can be buried at the foot of a tree.*

Ma'at: The pillar of fire is established as it was ordained to be. All is accomplished, Atum. Of thy seed will beauty come to thee. Now you may sleep on the breast of thy beloved.

*She takes off the head-dress and puts away the crook and flail. Taking his hands, she leads him to the bed and they lie down together. When they have rested they should again share their bodies with each other, for themselves alone, the Lord and Lady of Creation.*

# The Pathworking

You are conscious of yourself as a bodiless entity floating in a
starry void. Below you is a new, young and vibrant world. It has
been called into being by a God. He, too, is new-born in many
ways and this is the first of his creations. But although he has
created something beautiful and fair to see, with plant and animal
life abounding and the beginning of human life, he, Atum, is
alone with no other of his kind.

He floats in the void and you can hear his thoughts, feel his
loneliness and understand his pain. He awoke but a few aeons
ago and began his work of creation. This occupied him for a long
time, for he wished to make things perfect. When it was finished
he looked upon his work and admired it. Then he saw that the
animals and the people all had mates, ones they could love and be
with and with whom they might create more of their own kind.
But he, Atum, had no one.

You can hear the despair in his soundless voice and reach out to
him, calling him by name: 'Atum, Atum, Atum Ra.' At first he
cannot hear you, then as you draw astral flesh about you he sees
a vast silvery shape begin to take form. First a vast pair of scales
forms and behind them your own shape, a beautiful woman in
diaphanous robes. Long black hair floats around you as if it were
drifting on an unseen tide. About your brow gleams a golden
diadem, a snake rearing its head to strike.

You speak to the young God, telling him you are Ma'at, the
giver of truth and justice, that you come from beyond the void
from a place beyond time itself where the Gods that form the Gods
of this cosmos have their being. He asks for help and you offer
him knowledge beyond what he has at this moment, the secret of
his own androgynous being. Atum carries within himself his own
female self, the higher and more subtle part that still sleeps,
unawakened as yet to the power of Godhood.

Under your instruction the God becomes aware of this inner
self. You open his eyes and show him Tefnut. She is young and as
slender as a Nile reed, with hair as black as the void about her.
Her eyes are closed in sleep and her lashes lie upon her cheek like
black crescents. Her mouth smiles as she dreams and waits to be
called forth from her nest in the heart of Atum. Her breasts rise
up like firm pomegranates and her skin is like the dawn sky,
flushed with sleep. Her belly curves with promise and the jewel
between her thighs lies hidden beneath curls of ebony. Her legs
are graceful and her feet like tiny birds curled beneath her. All
beauty is found in Tefnut, sister, daughter and wife to Atum the
creator.

With care and gentleness you instruct Atum in the magic of bringing forth his beloved from within. Slowly she manifests, still sleeping, her body transparent for she is not yet fully awakened. Her beauty arouses Atum's desire and the God becomes a man in full pride. Tefnut floats in the void and the stars can be seen through her body. Atum holds her narrow hips in his hands and enters Her. Linked together the Gods are one and the seed of Atum flows into his beloved like a stream of silver stars. The child that will become Shu the God of air begins to form instantly and the body of Tefnut becomes more solid as her pregnancy grows. Her eyes open and she looks upon Atum and smiles.

The child flows from her body with ease and settles against her breast. The one became two and are now three. You release the astral matter of your body and become formless again. The three Gods recede as you withdraw from them. There is a sound of rushing wind, the pull of a power vortex and your own physical body receives you safely once more.

# Ritual 11

# THE RITE THAT IS LEFT UNDONE

## The Programme

This is the last of the rituals, the last in more ways than one. It is a ritual to do only once in your lives, and a ritual to be very, very sure about before you do it. Be sure of yourselves and your commitment to each other because once done, it cannot be undone. However I do ask you to understand and believe me when I say that no matter what may happen to your relationship in the future, the love and joy that has been shared can never really die – it remains held in its own time, perfect and whole and without blemish. This is true of everything we do that is beautiful and good: whatever we may do afterwards, that deed of beauty and goodness is not tarnished but remains as a symbol of what we can be if we so choose.

As we grow older the sexual content of our bonded lives grows less but the love burns just as brightly after another fashion. Each life we live brings us into different situations, pairs us with other partners and gives us other relationships, though sometimes the bonding is so strong that across the centuries one soul will call to another to join it and be together once more. The ultimate destination of humankind is Godhood, and that will only be possible when every atom of the body of the divine Osiris is brought together. In that multiple blending of spirit all relationships will be infinite and entwined. This is what is meant by the statement that in heaven there is no giving or taking in marriage. There will be no need of marriage as we know it, for humanity will be whole and part of the One.

To love unselfishly and without demand is rare, and there are those who cling to what they know and will not make that one tiny step beyond knowingness into full beingness. It will come, but we as a lifewave are as yet young and wayward. To let those we have loved leave us and go on without us or to go ourselves

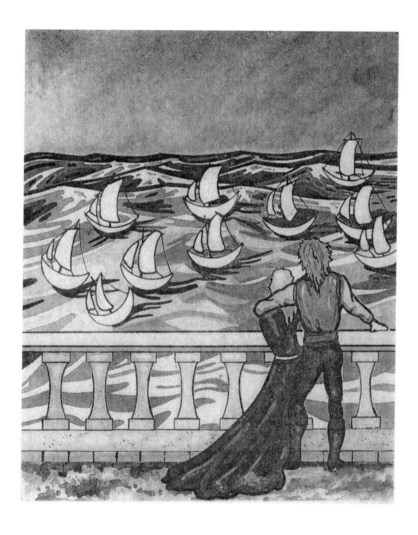

*Figure 24:* Happiness and Contentment *(Anthony Clark, from The Servants of the Light Tarot)*

into the unknown and not look back is hard, but if we trust and take that first step we will find that our fears were unfounded and that far from losing we will have gained much more.

This is a ritual of the understanding of death and the need to let go. It is at once a farewell and a promise of greeting when the time is right. Because we cannot know the moment of our death the ritual is left without an ending: it is the Rite that is Left Undone.

What is such a ritual doing in a book of sexual magic? It is here because the power you use to set and lock the 'future' spiritual event comes from the sexual power you will use now. For this the sphere of work on the Tree of Life is Kether, the point of manifestation, and this manifestation works both ways, both to come *into* life or to *depart* from life into a higher existence.

I have written in another book* about the need to work a Death Path, one that will begin to work when the point of death is reached. It will take you across to a place you have planned yourself and where you can rest. This ritual is designed to bless and hallow the bond between you so that whatever may happen later in this life or in future incarnations you will be able to draw upon the happiness and the joy you shared, and not be burdened by any bitterness or blame. If you should meet in a distant time you will recognize the bond you shared but it will not interfere with the life you will then be living. In short, this ritual will make you aware of the vast scope of *love* within the cosmos and of the fact that you will never really lose touch with each other or with the special feeling that you have enjoyed.

If you believe in reincarnation you must also understand that down through the centuries you have had, and will have, other wives, husbands, lovers and children. But you never 'lose' them – again and again your paths will cross and the love well up between you. My own two children were 'called' for, recognized and welcomed as they took their first breath. We have all been together many times and we know we will be together again. The intensity with which I love my family in this incarnation is the intensity with which I love those other souls who have been my children before.

This is a part of the doctrine of rebirth that people seldom think right through. They assure each other that they will be together again but they do not always realize that they have said the same thing to other loves. The love we feel for the families we have in this life is the same love we feel for every family we belong to throughout our many times on Earth. To bless and hallow each love we enjoy is to raise that love to something higher and purer. That is the intention of this ritual.

* *Highways of the Mind*, The Aquarian Press, Wellingborough, 1987.

There are no God forms for this ritual: you are your own Gods. Kether is the Great Simplicity and has no need of symbols or forms. It is everything and everything is Kether. The only exercise you need to do is to write down in a small notebook memories, both happy and sad, of your life so far with your partner. Tell them of your love for them and what it has meant to you. Search out poems that say what you feel, find a flower to press inside the pages, stick in pictures that you find especially beautiful or moving about love or family or life. At the end of the week wrap the notebook up like a present and exchange it with that of your partner.

Arrange a small table with a white cloth and a large white candle surrounded with flowers. Place there a chalice of wine and some bread on a plate with a small saucer of salt beside it, a little incense if you wish and two roses. Place chairs covered with clean white sheets facing the altar and place cushions on the floor to raise your feet. Do not wear robes, but ordinary clean clothes. Place as a focal point on the altar a symbol that has meaning for you both – a mother statue, an ankh, a cross, the lingam, anything you choose.

# The Rite that is Left Undone

## Sphere = Kether. Keynote = The Understanding of Love in the Cosmos.

*The little altar is set up in another room, but the ritual will begin in the bedroom with the physical coming together. This is because the energy of the sexual act is needed to fuel the ritual that follows. Do not be taken in by the simplicity of the ritual, for it is not simple in its effect.*

*Prepare your bed as for the other rites with clean sheets sprinkled with sweet herbs and flower petals. The woman sits on the bed with a cushion beneath her feet as in the Calling Forth in the first ritual. The man sits or kneels before her. He takes her feet in his hands.*

**Man:** You walk in beauty as do all women. As you touch the earth it gives forth its power. In you I worship the earth.

*He clasps her knees and lays his head upon them.*

When you kneel before the Goddess, She manifests in you. You are the garment of Isis. In you I worship her.

*He parts her knees and bends forward to kiss her vulva.*

You are the gate of life, the giver of form. Without you my life force cannot exist. In you I become a lord of life.

*He kisses each breast and holds them in his hands.*

You are the giver of nourishment both earthly and spiritual. You feed me as a mother and pleasure me as a Goddess. Within you I am both child and king.

*He kisses her mouth.*

You are the embodiment of the word, for from you come all things that live, move and have their being. You are love, you are completion, you are woman.

*He rises and they change places. Do not hurry, take it slowly. The woman takes the man's feet in her hands.*

Woman: You walk in strength and in that strength I am enfolded. As in the ancient days you are the power of the sun. By you, I as the earth am made fruitful.

*She clasps his knees and looks into his face.*

When you kneel before that which is divine, your spirit reflects that divinity. With you I worship the divine.

*She parts his knees, takes his phallus in her hand and kisses it.*

You are the holder of the life force. Without you I cannot form life, with you I am a maker of forms.

*She places both hands on his breast.*

You are my shield and my protection, my source of comfort and my joy.

*She kisses his mouth.*

You speak the word that I become and together we are the creators of all things. I fold my inner power around the rod of life and call you king to my queen.

*He lifts her up and together they lie down. They should look upon each other as two divine beings who are about to create a new point of manifestation. As they come together sexually they must hold the thought that they are part of the whole cosmos, and the cosmos a part of them. They represent all those they have loved and will love in the future. Let the power from that love build up within and retain it in the sexual centres for use in the ritual.*

*Rest and lie quietly, then get up, wash and dress and go in to begin the ritual. As you go through it let the power within flow in a steady stream through the heart, solar and sexual centres out to the Oneness of All.*

## Ritual

Man: You are my love, you are my companion, you are woman. I offer myself to you as your love and your companion. I ask in love for the gift of your body, as I will, in love, offer the gift of mine.

Woman: I will take the gift offered and offer mine to you. Enfold and protect me, as I will enfold and empower you. Take my hand and my gift, become the king of this land and this temple which is my body and together we will become as Gods.

*Hand in hand they approach the altar. Light the candle and the incense, then bow slightly and walk to your chairs and sit. Meditate on the other rituals you have done, on your life together and on what your future might hold. When you feel the time is right, continue with the ritual. The woman rises and salutes the altar with upraised hand.*

*Woman:* I invoke the presence of that which is in all things. Without form it moves upon the face of eternity. With a woman's power I invoke thee. With a woman's love I invoke thee. With a woman's hope I invoke thee. Come, divine presence, that we may be one with thee.

*The man rises and salutes the altar.*

*Man:* I invoke that which created the universe and ensouled it with itself. With a man's power I invoke thee. With a man's strength I invoke thee. With a man's pride I invoke thee. Come, thou nameless and divine one.

*The woman comes to the altar and raises the chalice.*

*Woman:* Enter this chalice, symbol of my womanhood. Let me give thee form in the wine it contains.

*She waits with head bowed for a moment, then replaces the chalice and takes up the bread.*

Enter this bread, symbol of the earth's gift, and pass into our bodies.

*She waits a moment, then replaces the bread and takes up the salt.*

Enter this salt that we may know thee in the elements. We behold ourselves in thee and in our mortal bodies we see thy divinity.

*The man rises and comes to the altar. He takes up the candle.*

*Man:* Enter this light, symbol of inner fire, that it may give thee physical fire.

*He replaces the light and takes up the incense.*

Enter this offering of incense that I may honour thee.

*He replaces the censer and takes up the roses.*

Enter these flowers that we may see thy gifts and praise thee.

*The man turns to the woman.*

*Man:* Thou art woman, and the power of form is yours. The cup holds thy power. Will you share with me your power of form? The power of growth is yours, and the bread is the symbol of growth. Will you share with me your power of growth? The power of the moon is yours, and the salt of your tears is its symbol. Will you share with me your tears?

*The woman offers him wine, then drinks. She offers him bread dipped in salt, then takes some for herself.*

*Woman:* Take unto thyself this portion of my power. Thou art man, and the power of life is yours. The candle holds its fire. Will you share with me that fire? The power of strength is yours, and the incense offers that strength. Will you share with me your strength? The pride of a man is that he can understand beauty. Will you share with me your understanding?

*The man takes the candle and circles the woman's head with it. He*

*replaces it and, taking up the censer, he censes her. Then he replaces the
censer and gives her one of the roses, keeping one for himself.*

*Man:* I share with thee my man's power, my fire and my strength
– now and in time to come.

*The couple return to their chairs, turn them to face each other and sit.
The man looks into the eyes of the woman.*

*Man:* I know you of old, you are part of me, part of my spirit
and my heart. We have shared our minds and bodies in love. Part
of me will be with you always. In lives to come I will feel your
presence in the world and seek you out. If I cross the Styx before
you I will be there to greet you. What we have shared will become
part of the divine being as we, in time, will become a part of it.

*Woman:* We two are one, you are a part of my spirit and my life.
Whatever the future holds for us this time will be kept bright and
whole. In lives to come I will know your face and remember what
we have shared. If I must go ahead I will wait to welcome you. If
you cross the Styx before me I will let you go on into the light. My
body will grieve but my soul will sing for you. What we have will
always exist.

*Man:* For all that you have brought into my life, I bless you. For
what we still have to share, I bless you. For what will be in the
future, I bless you.

*Woman:* For what you are as a man and as a being, I bless you.
For what you have given to me with your body, I bless you. For
what we will always have, I bless you.

*Man:* In all things, in all times, in all ways I will be with you. If I
must let you go, it will be in the knowledge that nothing can really
part us as spirits.

*Woman:* Let us pledge ourselves that in future lives and in other
relationships we will recall the love we now have.

*Both turn to the altar.*

*Man:* So it shall be and so we pledge. In token of this pledge I
……. *(his name)*

*Woman:* I ……. *(her name)*

*They walk to the altar and place their linked hands upon it.*

*Both:* Do offer up our love in this life to the will of the divine.
We ask a blessing on all those who have in the past been close to
us in love, and upon those who will be close to us in future lives.

*They kiss and share the last of the wine.*

*Man:* This ritual is not to be finished. It will go on forever.

*Woman:* It will go on . . .

# The Pathworking

You stand together hand in hand on the top of a high hill. It is twilight and the first stars are out. You can feel your love for each other as a tangible thing, an aura that surrounds you with warmth and light. Overhead shines a single bright star and as you watch there emerges from it a thread of light that drops towards the earth. Nearer and nearer it comes and soon you see that it is a broad stream of mist filled with points of light.

Down and down it drops until it is right above you. Now you see that the points of light are people. They are of all races, ages, and types, men, women and children. The stream touches the earth and the forms begin to flow past you. Each one looks for a moment into your face and smiles then passes on into the gathering night.

Many of them you do not know, but some cause a recognition to wake within you. Some are instantly known and you smile, laugh and wave, others look at you and then look away either in sadness or despair. Each one of them is from your past incarnations, people you have loved and been close to in your other lives. Here are wives, husbands, parents, children, brothers and sisters. To some you may be able to give a name, others are just faces. But as they pass you bless them, each and every one of them, for at some time in the past they have meant much to you.

You will see children once born to you, lovers from whom you may have been separated by disaster, death or chance. Parents who once held you in their arms and siblings you have played with long ago. They pass into the night and are gone but the love that has been reawakened in you remains. You understand more clearly that you can never be parted from someone you have loved, that when in the subtle realms you can recall their faces and your time together at will.

They have all passed and for a while there is nothing, but still you wait. Then comes another stream of forms, but now they pass to the other side of you. In this new river of life you see faces that are new to you. They are those who will come into your life in the future, in lives yet to come. They look hopefully at you, as if asking you to remember them when you meet. Again, let your love flow out to them and let them know that you will carry their images in your heart.

Once again the night swallows them up and there are just the two of you together in your own time. Try to understand that you will never be really separated, never lost from each other, just as you are never lost from those you have seen. All are One.

# EPILOGUE

Men and women are wonderful, beautiful beings, and when they come together sexually they are powerfully creative. This power can be used in many ways and for many purposes: to create situations, ideas, changes in your life, books, poetry, paintings, and of course children.

Sex is neither dirty nor sinful. It has been said, 'There is no part of me that is not of the Gods' – it is true, believe it. Your body is not something to be despised, beaten, flagellated, or abused by drugs. It is a temple housing a God, and that God is *you*. It has a string of natural power sources called chakras, centres going from the top of the head to the feet. Each of these centres is a concentration point for a different kind of power ranging from wisdom to emotion, body energy to communication. The most powerful of all is the sexual centre, and this is because its power is that of raw creation, the universal urge to 'make' something manifest. The universe is ever becoming, always creating, eternally manifesting, and you are a part of that, a minute cog in the machinery of the universe. Sex keeps that cog oiled.

Touching your lover's body or touching your own is not a sin: it's nice, healthy and what hands were made for, touching things. Self-abuse as applied to masturbation should be taken out of the language. Believe me, it will *not* make you blind, send you mad or make your hands hairy. Neither will it make you impotent. For some people it is all they will ever have in the way of sex. It is nicer with two, but if that is not possible you do not have many options.

The old idea that sex was something you did under several blankets, with the light out and never on a Sunday is as dead as the proverbial dodo. On the other hand promiscuity is not the thing either: sleeping around with Tom, Dick and Harry (or for that matter with Phyllis, Betty and Marje) is not a good idea in the present sexual climate. This book is for people who are:

1) Trained magicians, initiates, or at least fairly on in their training.
2) Bonded couples, lovers, married couples or solidly-based working magical partners.

It is *not* for those who have just picked up the book for kicks: kicked is just what they may get from the powers they awaken. Nor is it a guide book for swapping parties, office parties, or self-styled high priests and priestesses to use as a means of getting to know new members of their magical group. I have been a magician for too long not to be aware of how this book could be misused, so I have built in what might be termed 'guard dogs' to each ritual. Some people will spot them, others may not, but they are there. Use them for the wrong purpose and I guarantee you will not do it again. You can read into that statement what you will!

I am sure it will not have escaped your notice that all these rituals are written for heterosexuals. This is not to be interpreted as a criticism of homosexuals. I have friends in both areas of the gay community, and the rituals do not need specification. If you wish to amend them it is merely a matter of changing titles or a few words here and there.

To members of the Church who will hate this book on sight I would say this: *for the Love of your God and our Goddess,* come into the twenty-first century and try to understand that we in the occult world are no threat to you. Nor do we wish you harm in any way. Do not bring back the burning times in thought if not in deed. Do not class us all by the few, as we do not class all of you by the Inquisition.

'It is my commandment that ye love one another.'

# BIBLIOGRAPHY

Atkins, J., *Sex in Literature*, Panther, 1970.
Begg, E., *The Cult of the Black Virgin*, Arkana, 1985.
Berzin, B., *Sex Songs of the Ancient Letts*, University Books Inc., 1969.
Braddock, B., *The Bridal Bed*, Corgi, 1964.
Chia, M., and King, M., *The Taoist Secrets of Love* (2 vols), 1981.
Comfort, A. (ed), *More Joy of Sex*, Quartet Books, 1974.
Crawley, E., *The Mystic Rose*, Spring Books, 1927.
Cutner, H., *Sex Worship*, wartime edition.
Douglas, N., and Slinger, P., *Sexual Secrets*, Destiny Books, 1979.
Evola, J., *The Metaphysics of Sex*, East West Publications, 1983.
Fortune, Dion, *The Esoteric Philosophy of Love and Marriage*, The Aquarian Press, 1957.
Goldberg, B., *The Sacred Fire*, Jarrold, 1937.
Graves, R., and Patai, R., *Hebrew Myths: The Book of Genesis*, McGraw-Hill, 1963.
*Greek and Roman Erotica*, Miller Graphics, 1982.
Hall, Nor, *The Moon and the Virgin*, Harper and Row, 1980.
Harding, E., *Women's Mysteries*, Rider, 1971.
Horner, T., *Sex in the Bible*, Chas E. Tuttle and Co., 1974.
Humana, C., and Wang Wu, *The Chinese Way of Love*, CFW Publications, 1982.
King, F., *Sexuality, Magic and Perversion*, Spearman, 1971.
Koltuv, B.B., *Book of Lilith*, Nicholas Hays Inc., 1986.
Lannoy, R., and Baines, H., *The Eye of Love*, Rider, 1976.
Meltzer, D., *Birth*, North Point Press, 1981.
Neumann, E., *Amor and Psyche*, Bollingen, 1977.
Norbu, N., *Dzogcher, The Self-Perfected Way*, Arkana, 1989.
Patai R., *The Hebrew Goddess*, Ktav Publishing House, Hoboken, 1967.
– *The Gates to the Old City*, Avon, New York, 1980.
Rattray Taylor, G., *Sex in History*, Thames and Hudson, 1953.
Schwartz, H., *Tales from the Smokehouse*, Hurtig Press, 1974.

Scott, G.R., *Phallic Worship*, Panther, 1970.
Seltman C., *Women in Antiquity*, Pan Books Ltd, 1956.
Shuttle, P., and Redgrove, P., *The Wise Wound*, Gollancz, 1978.
Stone, Merlin, *Ancient Mirrors of Womanhood* (2 vols), New Sybelline Books Inc.
– *When God was a Woman*, New Sybelline Books Inc.
Tannahill, R., *Sex in History*, Abacus, 1980.
Thompson, W.I., *The Time Falling Bodies Take to Light*, Rider/Hutchinson, 1981.
Walker, B., *The Women's Encyclopedia of Myth and Secrets*, Harper and Row, 1983.
Wall, O.A., *Sex and Sex Worship*, C.V. Mosby Co., St Louis, 1922.
Wilson, C., *The God and the Labyrinth*, Granada, 1970.

# USEFUL ADDRESSES

Books, incenses, oils, and occult supplies are available from the following:

## United States

**Ancient Ways**
4075 Telegraph Avenue, Oakland, CA 94609
Phone: (510)653-3244, Fax: (510)653-3269, E-mail: ancways1@aol.com

**Arsenic & Old Lace**
318 Harvard Street #10, Brookline, MA 02146
Phone: (800)279-7785, Internet: www.arsenic.com

**Enchantments**
341 East 9th Street, New York, NY 10003
Phone: (212)228-4394
Send $3, check or money order, for their complete mail-order catalog.

**Mystickal Tymes**
127 South Main Street, New Hope, PA 18938
Phone/Fax: (215)862-5629, E-mail: mystymes@voicenet.com
Internet: www.mystickaltymes.com

**The Sphinx Metaphysical Bookstore**
1510 Piedmont Avenue, Suite H, Atlanta, GA 30324
Phone: (404)875-2665 or (800)801-4013 (pin# 9343) Fax: (404)875-3372
E-mail: sphinxbk@mindspring.com
Internet: www.mindspring.com/~sphinxbk

# United Kingdom

**Fantasy Candles**
"Glanrhyd," Llanfair, Clydogau, Nr. Lampeter, Wales, UK
Candles for all occasions

**Paul Hardy**
31 Gateacre Road, Owestry, Shropshire SY11 1DN, UK
Magical paintings/artwork

**Magis Books**
98 Ashby Road, Loughborough, Leicestershire, LE11 9AF, UK
New, rare, and secondhand books

**Mysteries of Albion**
122 High Street, Delabole, Cornwall PL33 9AJ, UK
Insences, oils, wands, staffs, and all magical and shamanic equipment

**Dusty Miller**
The Last Pagan Cudgel Master
21 Grange Road, Strood, Kent ME2 4DA, UK
Live wood staffs of all kinds, made in the traditional way, dating back some 1,000 years.

**Osiris**
19 Heath Road, Twickenham TW1 4AW, UK
Egyptian statues, paintings, posters

**The Sorcerer's Apprentice**
4/8 Burley Lodge Road, Leeds LS6 1QP, UK
For all occult supplies

**Watkins Bookstore**
19 Cecil Court, London WC2N 4EZ, UK
New, rare, and secondhand books

# INDEX

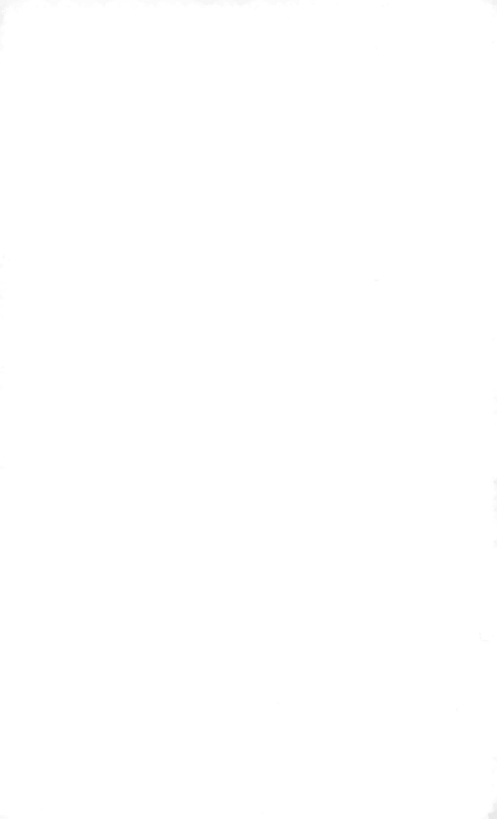